The Diagnosis Diaries

The Diagnosis Diaries

How one woman learned the uncertainty of her future and started living life to the fullest

Susan Kelley

ISBN: 9798379332396

For William, the best husband, the best friend, and the most positive person I've ever met. Congratulations on excelling at a job you never applied for—that of caregiver.

This book is dedicated to the millions of people dealing with chronic diseases. Stay positive, keep the faith and never ever give up.

Because if I tell the story, I control the version. Because if I tell the story, I can make you laugh, and I would rather have you laugh at me than feel sorry for me. Because if I tell the story, it doesn't hurt as much. Because if I tell the story, I can get on with it.

—**Nora Ephron**

TABLE OF CONTENTS

So often in life, things that you regard as an impediment turn out to be great, good fortune.

—Ruth Bader Ginsburg

INTRODUCTION

I don't know what the answer is!
I've decided to chronicle my new health situation without knowing the outcome—aka "what the answer is." (My mother's made-up words and stock phrases became part of our family vocabulary growing up, and this one in particular drove me crazy: "I don't know what the answer is!") *Her* final answer was that she was in her late nineties and had colon cancer. I am past the age of 70, stressed from taking care of her, but otherwise consider myself happy, active, and healthy. Then, out of nowhere, I've started to experience falls and muscle weakness in my legs and *I don't know what the answer is*, but more importantly, neither does my doctor.

My mother died last April, six months ago, at the age of 99 and one month. I was there; otherwise I would not believe that this force of nature had left the planet. She had remained in remarkably good health till age 96, did not need glasses following cataract surgery at age 84, still drove till 95—if you could call it that—and still utilized her enormous power over me although she no longer had it. She did her daily crossword puzzles, read constantly, prayed the rosary and attended Sunday Mass, and never missed her weekly hair appointment. I figured this was not bad for aging.

Her longevity left me with the unrealistic expectation that I myself would glide healthfully through life well into my nineties. This was calculated on my father's age at his untimely death at 84 and my mother's overdue demise. Fifteen years, split the difference, and I'd be healthy and active until at least age 91.

I expect that by the end of this story, I will know the answer, and I hope it's a happy one that can be fixed. For me, that chapter remains to be written. As the author of six published books, I remain as besotted with words and storytelling as I have ever been—though for the first time the subject is not one I would ever have chosen or imagined. But if I can weave my words into something worth reading and if I can help even one person in a similar situation, it will be worth it. I may even help myself as this story unfolds, because I have no idea what lies ahead or where this frailty came from.

PART ONE

Chapter 1
THE SITUATION

October 2018

One year ago exactly, in the fall of 2017, my husband and I were in Italy, traveling by train, something we have done often in the past 20 years—except for 2016, the year he had the terrible accident. More on that later. We were switching to a commuter train at Siena station. I was holding a tote bag in one hand, and in the other a framed art print—a gift for the people we were visiting.

Bill boarded first with the suitcase and I was to follow, but I had difficulty climbing the steep stairs of the old InterCity with no free hand to hold onto the grip bar. I fell forward, cutting my lower left leg on the corroded metal stair, lost my balance, and tumbled backward two stairs and onto the concrete platform, cracking the back of my head so hard, I saw stars.

I was dead. I opened my eyes in *heaven* to numerous people gathered around me, shouting in Italian *"Mamma mia, chiama un'ambulanza!'* (Call an ambulance? Was someone hurt?) I could hear Bill calling out my name from the top of the stairs of the train car but I was unable to answer—dead people can't talk. That was the beginning of my *situation.*

It's been over a year since I told my primary care doctor about my leg weakness and that fall off the train. She suggested at the time that I should go for an assessment of my balance.

The physical therapist, conveniently located downstairs from and recommended by my Pilates studio teacher, administered a few simple tests and said my balance was okay. I related the story about my backward tumble off the train in Italy. "Hmmm," he said. "I always wanted to go to Italy." The prescription from the doc said "Check for balance," and he did, and I passed. No PT needed. See you later. Return to square one.

Months go by. Our condo in Sarasota, Florida has no interior stairs, but there are stairs to the pool. Who uses the pool anymore? We've both had skin cancers. There are 11 stairs to the garage. They have become increasingly difficult to climb, especially when I return with shopping bags from Whole Foods. But I have no problem descending the stairs.

In the fall we return to Italy, as we always do. Bill is an artist and I am a writer; we both work in Florence. This has been our modus operandi for almost 20 years. Once, we rented a beautiful condo for four years. Now we go for three months every autumn.

This October in Florence, I feel as if Bill is dragging

me around. I hang tightly to his arm as we navigate the cobblestone streets and sidewalks with loose bricks. I have become the "albatross," but we are managing, and he is not complaining. We have always been big walkers; we don't drive in Florence; we don't even have a car. We walk everywhere. But now it feels like I have sacks of potatoes tied onto each of my thighs, making walking tedious. And then a strange and frightening thing happened. We were with some friends at a restaurant, and suddenly I experienced flashes of light on the sides of both eyes. The next morning I had small dark spots and squiggly lines floating across my vision.

I called my ophthalmologist in Sarasota, who explained they were called flashes and floaters, and it could be a torn retina issue. He told me to have it checked out immediately in Florence. I made an appointment at Correggi Teaching Hospital, where mercifully they spoke perfect English. Following a thorough eye exam, they informed me there was no retinal damage. The rest of our Tuscan sojourn was uneventful, but the black spots in my vision persisted.

———

We arrived in Chapel Hill, NC for Christmas. My daughter and husband are both physicians. "Mom," Dr. Daughter says, "why can't you get up the stairs?"

Husband Dave is an orthopedist also at UNC. He suggests I see a colleague in Sarasota. After continuing our holiday travels to Boston to see the rest of the family, I came home to Sarasota and made an appointment with the orthopedist.

January 2019

The symptoms came on slowly, manifesting primarily as muscle weakness in my quadriceps. I returned to my primary care physician. "I'm having difficulty walking up stairs. I can't get up from a chair without pushing myself off. It's beyond difficult to get up from the toilet." I'm over 70, but this is not considered old here in the retirement capital of the United States: I'm a kid! Doctor orders complete blood labs.

It would be another year before we would find answers. And now it begins, numerous visits to doctors and specialists, a series of tests, speculations and ambiguity. I am familiar with doctor offices, labs, and the hospital, having spent the last five years taking my mother on constant rounds of appointments.

We have dinner with some young friends. She shows me her results of cool sculpting. I make an appointment for a consult and find out it will cost $3000 for the procedure including follow-up. Okay, a flat stomach will help me feel better. I could easily afford this with the recent bequest from my mother's estate.

———

At the end of January I get a call from my primary care physician's office from a non-medical person. Monday: "Your bloodwork came back and all is fine." I sigh a sigh-of-relief.

"See," Bill says. "It's all in your head."

Second call two days later from same office with same information. "Your bloodwork came back and all is normal." "Thanks," I say again.

The following Monday morning yet another call: "Your bloodwork came back. "Yes, I know, I've had two calls. Thank you." "You have rheumatoid arthritis." "What?" "Sorry, hon," says the office person who is neither a doctor nor a nurse nor anyone I have ever met. Bill and I just completed our morning two-mile walk. "Well, let's face it," he says, "we're over 70 and many athletes have arthritis." We drink our coffee and eat our homemade gluten-free, almond flour, blueberry muffins that I just baked.

I turn on the computer and Google rheumatoid arthritis. WOW. It's bad! I'll be in a wheelchair within the year. Next day is my appointment with son-in-law's orthopedist colleague.

Chapter 2
TRYING TO FIND THE DIAGNOSIS

I'm distraught and almost run over a man and his dog on the way to the doctor's office. While driving, I make a solemn commitment to God. I will not do cool sculpting—even though my much younger friend looks fabulous—if I don't have RA. What the fuck! My first deal with God in a very long time.

Orthopedist looks at bloodwork with elevated levels of muscle enzymes. He does a series of physical tests. "You don't have any signs of RA," he says, but says he thinks it's a form of myositis and recommends I see a rheumatologist and or neurologist. This is not his field. I have never heard of myositis. At least he did not say cancer. And it's not rheumatoid arthritis. Thank God for the man and his dog. They'll be safe now, should I pass them again on my way home.

He tells me the muscle enzymes are elevated and the rheumatoid factor was positive. Do I have any autoimmune diseases? Yes, I have psoriasis (long in remission), so this is why the rheumatoid factor came back positive.

Next appointment is with a young and seriously attractive—dressed in a running outfit with sneakers, and around the age of my children or younger—**neurologist.** He does some physical tests and concurs I do not have any signs of RA. He asks me to get up. I push myself from the armchair. He says it's not bad. At least I can shove myself up. I explain that I am unable to hop or skip. My feet won't come off the floor. "Why would you want to skip?" he asks. I attempt humor. "I won't be able to dance at weddings. My husband says this is a good thing." He laughs. *Why do I feel the need to entertain the doctor?* He tells me to come back in a few months if my symptoms don't improve.

On to the **rheumatologist**, who says my situation is "not normal." She orders bloodwork (17 vials), testing for about everything including Lyme disease, TB, probably beri-beri . . . who knows? When all come back normal, she orders an MRI of my thighs. "If it comes back showing Inflammation," she tells me, "you will need to get a muscle biopsy."

I don't really want to get my thigh cut open, but I call the recommended **neurosurgeon**, and the office tells me they don't do the procedure. This buys me time. I ask my primary care doc for two things: 1) a brain scan (Maybe I damaged my brain falling off the train and cracking open the back of my skull, which could also be related to my eye flashes); and 2) a script for Physical Therapy, which I hit with a vengeance—three times a week. The new and trendy privately owned for-profit PT has all the latest equipment.

It is close by and convenient. I commit to a heavy duty program, and in a short time I seem to be getting stronger.

Sat, May 4, 2019

I went in the pool yesterday and again today: water exercise is beneficial. Today Bill comes with me. Climbed up ladder stairs to get out, fell on top rough step, cut my leg, bleeding (not bad), and scraped the other. UGH. One step at a time. I would have walked out, but there was a kid with two blowup toys blocking the stairs. A little depressing; Band-Aids on both legs. At night I drink a glass of wine with dinner. I must have made a mistake and been optimistic. This is definitely NOT all in my head!

Back at Neurologist, who looks at bloodwork, chats, and does another series of tests.

Mon, May 6, 2019

Eleventh physical therapy session today. Still can't lift off the floor, hop, skip, or jump. Went to hospital for additional bloodwork ordered by rheumatologist. (Is she a vampire?) Also more at another lab Wednesday. She also requested a chest x-ray. I stood there looking at the order, which said, "Diagnosis: Shortness of breath." I do not have nor have I ever experienced shortness of breath. So I turned around, left without the x-ray, and called the office to ask why it was ordered. Have not heard back yet. I really am trying to get to the bottom of this. Asked lab person drawing blood what it was for: tuberculosis, hepatitis, muscle enzyme, Lyme disease . . .

Wed, May 8, 2019

I am committed to finding out what is causing the issue. I go to the second blood lab with the order. They take two vials and FedEx to California. Hope the results get back in a week so I can figure it all out. Next step I decide I *will* go for chest x-ray at Sarasota Memorial.

Fri, May 10, 2019   Lift Off

Today marks the end of four weeks @ 3x a week in Physical Therapy. I feel a lot stronger and no longer have a fear of falling. My balance is good.

I went on a series of sort of hopping from one square to another. Then therapist gave me hand weights. I was to squat as far as I could (not much), chest up, and swing weights back and then forward for momentum and try to hop with both feet. I've done this before, but today to no avail. My feet stick to the floor like they have been stapled.

Erin stands close by, first demonstrating, then coaching. On my third attempt, my feet miraculously moved about an inch off the floor. Everyone claps.

Erin asked if I thought I had come as far as I can. I said no. She suggests my problem is *"dead butt syndrome"* from sitting and writing all day—*"No-Ass-At-All"* she says, laughing. "Don't tell anyone I said this." My lips are sealed. Just want to be fixed. She could be right—I spent nine months sitting and writing a movie about Bill's accident. Definitely too much sitting.

Bill's Accident: Treatment for a Screenplay Based on True Events

William (Bill), a Boston-bred successful businessman turned professional artist, believes he has it all—a beautiful wife, loving children and grandchildren, and living the dream as an artist, splitting his time between his studios in Florence, Italy and Sarasota, Florida.

His perfect world is rocked, however, when he is involved in a horrific automobile accident. During a Stateside visit with family, Bill, a dynamic and gregarious painter, is riding as a passenger in the right rear seat of a professional car service and chatting amicably with the driver, when suddenly the car loses its brakes, begins to smoke, and catches on fire. Bill, engulfed in flames and without hesitation, instinctively dives out the rear passenger window of a still-speeding, burning automobile, lands on the side of a major interstate highway, and miraculously survives. The driver does not.

The Emergency Medical Service vehicle arrives on the scene and transports Bill to the Tampa General Hospital Burn Center. His wife, Susan (a writer), is home waiting for him when she gets the phone call. Susan rushes to the hospital, where she is met by a state trooper who ushers her to see her husband. His injuries are life-threatening: 35% of his body has suffered third-degree burns, which the doctor describes as "catastrophic." They believe he will require a minimum of four surgeries and at least three to four months in the hospital. His projected survival rate is less than 20%.

William and Susan are determined to beat the odds. With his indomitable will to live and to create more paintings, and to the amazement of his medical team, William survives two surgeries and is released from the hospital in a month. Following six more months of home rehabilitation and care, he is the featured artist at a major exhibition in Sarasota and subsequently returns to his beloved Florence to live and paint again. But the dynamic in the marriage is dramatically changed as Susan's role reverses to the dominant partner during Bill's recovery. By the end, the fierce ego that drives Bill's survival is also tamed and mellowed as he sees his incredible wife in a new light.

Chapter 3
EVERYONE'S AN EXPERT

Sun, May 12, 2019

Exhausted from physical therapy, at-home exercises, and Pilates, I give myself a gift of a 90-minute massage for Mother's Day, instead of staying home and hoping that my children might remember that they have a mother. I explain my aches and pains resulting from overwork and strength-training. I tell the therapist that all the results should be back when I have my Thursday appointment with the rheumatologist.

She mulls this over, and we have a brief discussion about PT. In the course of the massage, she shares that she thinks my issue may be Lou Gehrig's disease and that one of her clients has it and his symptoms of muscle weakness are similar to mine. So much for the "relaxing massage." I want to jump off the table and Google it to find out what my life expectancy is. I inhale a controlled breath and blow it out slowly as I tell her I am to see the doc, who will figure out the lab results. "Lou Gehrig's disease does not show up in bloodwork," she says definitively. "That's the problem." Everybody's a fucking expert!

I walk in my front door, down the hallway, and through our homey kitchen past Mother's Day flowers and strawberries dipped in chocolate, cheerfully displayed on the blue marbled granite island top, and go straight to the office computer. I don't seem to have the "Early signs and symptoms of ALS," which include: Hand weakness or clumsiness, slurred speech, or trouble swallowing. No trouble there; I've gained weight. Google is a terrifying tool.

Mon, May 13, 2019   Starting Week 5

Number 13 is good luck for me. I left my first husband on Friday, October 13, in another lifetime. Today, I manage a straight line of double hops—maybe eight. I worked up a sweat. It was my fourteenth PT. I have ten left, but going down to 2x a week this week. Aching thighs but hopeful. I am progressing, albeit slowly.

Tuesday, I played nine holes of golf with Bill. Feel like I'm on vacation. I was not as terrible as I was last week, our first time together. I actually had a few good shots, and he is very supportive.

Thurs, May 16, 2019

This week two PT sessions and feeling it particularly in hips. Still difficulty walking up stairs. I convince myself I must be patient. Today one hour Pilates. Marcie tells me I'm doing great but need to keep it up. When PT is over she suggests a personal trainer 2x a week to continue strengthening. Came home from Pilates and went to the condo pool for 20 minutes of running and hopping under water while wearing a protective hat. Beautiful day and no one in the pool. I live in a spa. I notice my skin on thighs is hanging and crepe-y. I need more toning.

Physical fitness is the first requisite of happiness.

– Joseph Pilates

At 4:30 today I return to the rheumatologist for answers. After blood testing for everything except pregnancy and HIV, one chest x-ray, and one brain scan, I will surely learn some reasons for the lack of muscle strength. I am extremely nervous. My Pilates instructor thinks it is from sitting and writing. "Sitting is the new smoking." Bill agrees. I don't have the strength for a chronic illness. My mother's only been gone a year. I want to enjoy life, my children and grandchildren.

Please God, good news and I will not do cool sculpting, I swear. I am sticking to our deal.

What if she tells me I have a few months to live? Polio? Cancer? I'll be too nervous to drive home. Bill wanted to come with me, and I said absolutely no way. Maybe there will be no news. In that case, I'll drop further tests and just try to keep strengthening.

Results:
Muscle enzyme up from 195 to 367. (Could this be a result of all the exercise?) This is way above the normal range of 26 -192

Chest x-ray normal
Kidney normal
Lyme Screen ok
Complete muscle panel: negative
TB negative
Lupus negative
Hep negative

Every test was negative, but rheumatoid factor came back positive and enzymes were elevated. Other than that, I was textbook healthy. Doc reiterates that the weak quadriceps muscles is not normal.

She insists on an MRI of one thigh. Could be inflammatory muscle disease, in which case she will possibly put me on methotrexate.

This is where I draw the line. No muscle biopsy, and I will not take methotrexate. (Yes, I Googled it.) I feel okay and am not in any pain.

Thurs, May 23, 2019

Today I am scheduled for the MRI of my left thigh. They are looking for inflammation. If MRI is normal, next step is nerve conduction study. If MRI is positive, back to the muscle biopsy and drugs.

I'm kind of at the end of my journey after four months of seeing all the doctors, getting the initial misdiagnosis of RA, six weeks in PT causing my CPK to increase to 367, chest x-ray, MRI of brain, and extensive bloodwork—all of which have come back negative. I am still not able to climb stairs normally, squat, skip, or get out of a chair without pushing myself up. The only diagnosis I still have is "myositis," unspecified. I am willing to try anything at this point. Neurologist told me to not exercise for two weeks, get another blood workup, and go see him. I cannot afford to not exercise for two weeks—I don't want to lose my new strength. I've worked very hard at PT for the past six weeks. Very frustrated at this point.

> I just had a call from the rheumatologist that MRI showed inflammation in some muscle groups, diffuse atrophy, and edema: Myositis. She refers me to a neurosurgeon.
> This is very scary.

Googling all afternoon. Causes and treatments. Muscle biopsy is the most accurate test for diagnosing myositis. A doctor identifies a weak muscle, makes a small incision, and removes a small sample of muscle tissue for testing. Muscle biopsy leads to a final diagnosis in most people with myositis.

Thurs, May 30, 2019

Meet with David, the head of PT, and tell him I am dissatisfied because after seven weeks of PT three times a week, I am stronger but the problem of not being able to get up is no better. I show him the MRI results. He gives me a major printout for daily exercise. I can even watch the video of how they are done.

Fri, May 31, 2019

Bone density results are in. I have osteopenia. Guess I should have taken the vitamin D I bought a year ago. Just purchasing it doesn't work. I suppose osteopenia can be stopped in its tracks with vitamin D, calcium, vitamin K, and weight-bearing exercises. I am not looking forward to the call re: the mammogram. Has not been a great year for me. By the way, I thought I was safe at my age but the tech told me—as she squished my right breast between two icy cold plates—that our chances for breast cancer increase as we age. Wow! *"No One Ever Told Me That!"* This was my mother's second-favorite expression. The reality is they did tell her, but like in the Simon & Garfunkel song "The Boxer": *A man hears what he wants to hear and disregards the rest.* In this case it was a woman—*Mm-mm-mm-mm-mm-mm!*

Thurs, Jun 6, 2019

Rheumatologist tells me the methotrexate would be for life. I have not yet scheduled a consult with the neurosurgeon for the biopsy. I'm going to NY next week for our anniversary and then back here in July and who knows what!!!!

Chapter 4
IS THIS WHAT ARE FRIENDS FOR?

So upset I e-mail my oldest friend who is an RN and relate my situation. She writes back:

I am remembering Bob's [her husband's] Myositis days.

Same type of symptoms as yours only his lack of muscle strength was in his upper body. He could not move his arms...He could not dress himself or take a shower or comb his hair. He was still working... Luckily, he had Dermatomyositis first.....which was thinning of the skin and bruising mostly on his hands and arms.

Rheumatologist gave him an Rx for Prednisone which he took.....big face, but he was mobile. And could get around...He still could not raise his arms. Ugh!

We went back to the rheumatologist. After a month of tests including Nerve Conduction study he was being weaned off the Prednisone and he started on the Methotrexate.....it was not a long protocol... We would see him every 2 weeks and there were blood tests to determine how well the Methotrexate worked...and it was a miracle drug...for this diagnosis.

Then the Throat Cancer. You need to line up an oncologist, because that's next. XO

At the last sentence, my jaw drops open. I don't even have similar symptoms as Bob, and I am now lining up an oncologist? My *friend* took special pride in developing her reputation as a medical expert. *Do friendships have a lifespan? Is this long one over?*

Fri, June 7, 2019

My longtime, trusted Pilates instructor thinks I may have a problem with my psoas muscle. She takes a video of me trying to do a wall squat and sends it to her strength expert friend in Ft. Myers. He immediately writes back that he thinks it *is* the psoas and he would like to help me. I schedule an appointment to drive an hour and a half to Ft. Myers. "Who is this quack?" Bill says after agreeing to go with me. I am excited at the prospect of finally getting to the bottom of this. I will see the guy in Ft. Myers and I will be okay.

Tues, June 11, 2019

The great trip to Ft. Myers for the cure did not turn out to be the Miracle of Fatima. The long, tiring drive was followed by a one-hour "consult" with an ancient guy (probably younger than me) who smelled old, unbathed, and seedy—along with two lovely girls who appeared to be his students. He was not interested in any pertinent info I brought with me, which included my x-ray, bloodwork showing elevated muscle enzymes, etc. He said my brain was not connecting to my muscles to do what they should. He said a muscle biopsy was ridiculous, gave me three exercises to do at home, and charged me $125. He would like to see me in a week. He did not say myositis or anything else. Sit less and exercise more. He stretched my psoas muscle.

On the way home I took a picture of a highway sign as we passed: "Port Charlotte," where my youngest brother had recently bought a house, and texted it to him: "Too bad you are not home for a visit. We had to drive to Ft. Myers." He asked why and I explained I was having some muscle issues. He jumped on the moment to add *his* diagnosis— which is what the singer Peter Frampton has....Inclusion Body Myositis. "It's untreatable," he texted.

I e-mail daughter doc and sports medicine husband re: trip to guru. I get this intelligent and caring response:

Yeah. These type of problems are often frustrating. I'm not sold on the Ft. Myers guy's psoas as the cause of all this but PT will only help you. Wish I had a better answer. Never did think it was RA. You have muscle weakness. That part is clear. The why is the unknown. Keep at the PT. If no improvement maybe reconsider the muscle biopsy. Ft. Myers guy is not a doctor (MD), he's a physical therapist and strength and conditioning expert. Not saying he's wrong but not a physician.

Today at PT, I got the results from a machine scan that measures body fat and muscle. I am way below normal with muscle on legs and arms. High fat, low muscle, and low water. The only thing halfway normal is my torso. I should probably shoot myself now. I am exhausted from exercising for the past three months and still have no muscle. Imagine what the test would have shown in the beginning? Probably zero strength.

My youngest brother of the Peter Frampton diagnosis and his wife were here for dinner when I was experiencing a recurrence of eye floaters and flashes. He told me he had recently read about a group of 18 patients in a small town in Huntersville, North Carolina, who had similar symptoms. One woman was diagnosed first: at age 27, she saw odd flashes of light and they were all diagnosed with a rare form of eye cancer. So comforting to have family around.

Feeling discouraged with my physical limitations. What if I do have some incurable disease? I need to write my will and choose a photo—preferably one of me much younger than I am now. This will be accompanied by a sterling obituary (I always lie about my age), which I will also write. *Is this too controlling?* I should probably address whether

I wish to be buried or cremated, as well as find a resting place for my remains.

Taking a long brutal look at myself, I am describing my frustration to Bill when he interrupts: "You can walk and you can fuck. What else do you want at age 75?" Happy Anniversary! I tell him that this type of remark is mansplaining: *The explanation of something by a man, typically to a woman, in a manner regarded as patronizing.*

www.merriam-webster.com/words-at-play/...Mansplaining is, at its core, a very specific thing. It's what occurs when a man talks condescendingly to someone (especially a woman) about something he has incomplete knowledge of, with the mistaken assumption that he knows more about it than the person he's talking to does.

I tell Bill that I feel anxious all the time. I tell him that I endured so much anxiety dealing with my mother that on more than one occasion, could feel physical changes occurring in my body. I tell him that the American Psychological Association defines anxiety as "an emotion characterized by feelings of tension, worried thoughts and physical changes like increased blood pressure."

I tell him that I cannot live for the next let's say fifteen years having to pull myself upstairs and not being able to get up from a toilet, particularly at airports—squatty potties! How did I get here? He comes over and delivers his big strong signature hug. He is smart, funny, positive, and self-assured. He makes me laugh—except when he pisses me off.

Wed, June 12, 2019

The American Standard Champion 4 right-height toilet is available in the color bone, which matches the rest of my master bathroom. It's billed as the leader in high-performance toilets and it complies with the height requirement set forth by the Americans with Disabilities Act, with a 16 ½-inch seat height. My first disabled purchase and installation.

Chapter 5
ATOMIC LEVEL STRESS

I should probably explain my relationship with my mother. When I was born, I was not matched by any parent app. It was a random choice on both sides. I was her second child. At about age three, I figured out that we didn't like each other, but we were stuck. Where would I go?

My older brother by seventeen months was her favorite, and I adored him. I was my father's favorite, and that was mutual for me. Unfortunately that left my four younger brothers with no particular family advocate, but they usually tried to get me to intercede on their behalf.

My mother was a tough cookie, born in the Bronx, a twin and the youngest of six. Following my father's death, she continued to live for eighteen years in Sarasota, twenty minutes by car from me. Over those years she sustained a number of falls, injuries, and surgeries, yet she made the most amazing recoveries I've ever witnessed. She was not a consenting adult when she transitioned to Assisted Living at age 96. Hospice even fired her twice—on one occasion, she told the doctor her impending demise was all a mistake, she had only eaten bad pudding, and he actually believed her. She returned to her temporary quarters and lived well for another year. Bill said she had more comebacks than Frank Sinatra.

Here's the thing: I was the only one in my family afflicted with my eternal mother.

She embodied criticism, dissatisfaction, and negativity, stridently, and always aimed at me—whereas my brothers (none of whom lived nearby) were in her word, "busy". Her behavior was a reflection of her own reality--she was unsatisfiable--but I took it personally, and in doing so I became a victim, always trying harder, always stressed, always failing to please. Her demands were constant and relentless, and everything was a battle: getting her to use a cane, a flat-out unwillingness to surrender her driver's license, her insistence on traveling across the country to visit one of her sons when she was well into her nineties, and refusing to accept a cellphone. The accompanying stress that fell to me was atomic level. This is not good for the immune system. I had purposely set out not to be anything like her. I always hoped my mother would magically turn into the mother I always wanted but never had. For so many people over the age of fifty or sixty, responsibility for an elderly parent is a major challenge, and their own health can easily be neglected and/or adversely affected. I was a poster child for this situation.

Sat, June 29, 2019

I asked the therapist if I should not be much better after three months of intensive physical therapy two to three times a week. She looked at me through forty-year-old eyes and said, "Yes, you should be better. Has your blood with muscle enzyme count come back yet?" I explained I had my annual physical in a few days and I would find out. Much is hinging on that outcome. Bloodwork done after trip to NY with no PT or Pilates for a week. Thinking they were way up last time because I was exercising so much.

I call the Neurosurgeon, who I still have not heard back from after weeks. Two days later I call again. I tell the receptionist or whatever she is that I want to make an appointment for a consult regarding a muscle biopsy. She responds slowly, spelling out his profession: "These are Neuro s u r g e o n s who do spinal surgery and not muscle biopsy of the thighs." I told her I had been referred by Dr. Rheumatologist, who has them ordered for patients all the time. Exasperated, she puts me on hold. Then, "Dr. K does do muscle biopsies." I ask if he will do a needle biopsy. Back on hold. No, it takes place in the hospital and is a three- to four-inch incision. Does not require overnight stay.

Mon, July 1, 2019

Today is the day of my annual physical and I will get the long-awaited results of my new bloodwork. As I'm getting dressed to leave for the appointment, the phone rings. The doctor did not feel well and went home for the day. Can we reschedule for next available appointment, which is several weeks away?

Wed, July 3, 2019

I cancelled the appointment on July 12 with the rheuma-tologist. No sense in going, since I decided not to have the required biopsy.

First appointment with personal trainer ($75 per hour; and highly recommended). She's good and she makes notes, displaying a level of involvement that makes me think she cares. I'm thinking the physical therapist is getting bored with me, as I don't really progress. The personal trainer tells me my spine is weak and "We're going to work on the spine as well as quads and glutes." We are a team! I am hopeful.

So far she is great. Started riding exercise bike fourteen minutes, five miles. Energizing.

Tues, July 9, 2019

Just had call from gynecologist's office. Pap test came back normal. Yipee. I'm taking this as a good sign, despite the eye floaters and my inability to get up from a toilet.

Fri, July 26, 2019

I am now going to PT 2x a week, Pilates once, and personal trainer once a week. Bill keeps telling me it's too much. I think I am getting stronger, although I am still unable to hop. I begin to notice the loose, hanging skin on my thighs and upper arms.

Going on vacation in one week. I arrive at PT for my 4pm confirmed training with David. "Hi, Susan, why are you here?" asks Cindi, the receptionist. "You don't have an appointment today." I zip open my purse, pull out my printed schedule, and point to today, Friday 4 pm, with David. She says: "I don't have you in my system. Who made the appointment?"

"You." I stand on the vibrating machine, and now it is 4:15 and I am meeting Bill and clients in an hour and a half, hopefully dressed and looking presentable. "You know what? That's okay, I'll leave. See you next week."

"Wait, David says he will see you." I am now conflicted and feel it is bad juju, but get coerced into the gym with David, who is clearly engrossed in helping another patient. *Always follow your instincts!*

New PT-in-training Kyla is smiling. "I have some new things for you to do today." Kyla is a very cheerful, energetic, very tall young woman of probably six feet. So we proceed. She has me do some sitting and getting up, and then she is laughing and says she wants me to pretend there is a line. Swing my arms forward holding weights and go up on my toes. She then removes the hand weights and tells me to keep swinging my arms and hop over the line. I try and can't do it. "I can't hop," I say. "That's why I'm here."

This is like her telling a patient to get out of the wheelchair and walk. "Come on, you can do it, you can do it, blah blah blah." Breaking a sweat, I fling my arms up for momentum and try with all my might to hop, and I make it an inch off the floor. "Okay, ten more," she pushes enthusiastically.

The second try does not end well. I simply cannot get

my feet off the floor, lose my balance in trying to do so, and twist my entire body to the left, falling and missing cracking my head by an inch. I lie there hurt and pissed off. Kyla is horrified and scared. "Come on, get up," she says as David leaves his client and rushes to the scene of the accident. "I have hurt my leg and I am unable to get up. That's the other reason I'm here. I cannot get up from the floor."

And so, after four months of training and finally feeling like I was getting stronger, I have a major setback. I am in severe pain. David tells me to come in for laser therapy every day before I leave for Boston. "It goes below the surface and helps to heal whatever happened." It has no effect, and I can hardly walk with the pain in my left leg and ankle. They bill my insurance for all of this. LIFE CHANGING!

Fri, August 9, 2019

Dear David,

It is now two weeks since my fall and I am no better: my left leg is still extremely painful and I am having difficulty walking. We are now in Boston for a month, and I can barely get around. If it doesn't improve in the coming week, I will have to see an orthopedic doctor here. I am so unhappy that this accident occurred. I had a specific appointment with you at 4pm on July 26, and when I arrived, you substituted a trainee who was too aggressive in her treatment and not as familiar with my limitations.

In my opinion this would not have happened if you had been working with me. I will keep you informed of my progress, but at the moment it is all beyond disappointing.   Susan Kelley

Dear Susan,

I too am disappointed you are continuing to have trouble with your left leg. When I last saw you prior to your departure from Sarasota, the lateral leg pain was able to be reproduced with palpation of the muscle along the outside of your leg, the peroneus longus, which had an irritable trigger point, which we then treated with the soft tissue laser and some soft tissue work. Fortunately, when we looked more closely at your left knee and tested for orthopedic involvement of your meniscus and patellofemoral (kneecap) joint, they both tested negative, and the tibiofemoral joint (main knee joint where the thigh and leg meet) was stable with testing (called the valgus and Varus stress test). So, that lateral leg pain should respond well to standard interventions for soft tissue irritability including massage, gentle stretching, and a progressive return to strengthening when tolerable. I hope your condition continues to improve, and I am happy to forward any information about it to any health care professional you feel you need to visit in the coming month to share any information you approve us to share. Please keep in touch, if you'd like to visit a PT up there, I can search the local zip code and recommend one from reviewing their profiles.David

Blah blah blah!!!!!!!!!!!!!!!!!!!!!!!

Chapter 6
TURNING UP THE MUSIC / RETURN TO ITALY

Maybe this will all just go away. At least I can walk. And so we return to our second home where we live a glorious and productive life.

October 2019 Week One

Walking with Bill in Rome, trying to be confident. All good. It's my fifth day of a two-month return visit to Italy. Rome for four days and then to Florence, our spiritual home.

This year the lovely top-floor-with-a-view apartment we usually rent is occupied until October 8. We accept a smaller one around the corner for five days. The realtor greets us warmly and upon entering, warns about a *passo pericoloso* (dangerous step) by the front door. We listen intently. There are an additional 22 stairs to a sleeping loft. The bathroom is also on the upper level. These are things that never would have bothered my old self. I pull myself up the stairs, one by one.

The next morning, as we are on our way to go out for a cappuccino, my husband waits by the front door. I walk quickly to meet him, forget about the step, trip, and fall.

Here, my vacation immediately changes. I hurt my right big toe and probably crack a rib as I land on the stair with my left side. "Are you okay?" my husband asks hopefully. The pain is excruciating. I pull myself together and out we attempt to go to get a coffee, but we don't get far.

I spend most of the day with an ice pack centered on right toe and additional ice on the affected left rib. I learn how to say "I broke my big toe" in Italian: Mi sono rotto l'alluce!

And so begins my time in Florence. Upon Googling, I find it will be three to six weeks for my recovery. Do I go to a doctor or hospital? No! There's a saying among Americans in Italy: Where do you go if you need medical attention? Answer: The airport. I break down and start to sob.

Besides taping the big toe to the one next to it, not much can be done. The rib will have to heal from the crack or bruise. The bone isn't sticking out, so I'll probably live.

The next morning Bill decides that perhaps we should cancel our upcoming planned spring trip in three months to Vietnam, Cambodia, and Thailand. Too strenuous!

Here's the thing. I am now 76 years old. I don't feel it and never thought it would happen to me, and I always deduct at least three years off my actual age, claiming my younger brother's birthday of 73—which is now also old.

But this year I have developed some form of myositis, making most toilets the ultimate challenge. My vision is also changing. It's the seventh inning, and I seem to be getting accident-prone.

I remember as a young child my grandmother talking about "maybe not being here," and I'd ask, "Where are you going?" I understand now—I am wondering the same thing.

November 2019   Second Tumble

This is the day my whole world turned upside down. We are back in our old apartment and have been enjoying autumn in Florence, despite my challenges of mobility. We've had visitors and we go out almost every night for dinner. This evening, it's cold and rainy as we walk through Piazza della Signoria to an art gallery nearby. We are meeting with the owner to discuss a possible exhibition of Bill's paintings for the coming year. Following our successful meeting, we have our usual aperitivo at Caffè Rivoire before heading to Buca Poldo for an early dinner. *Buca* in Italian means *hole*, so when Buca is in the name, it means the restaurant is in the basement or cellar. Outside dining is now closed for the season.

There is a long circular staircase to downstairs seating, where we have been dining for twenty years. This night is different because I am different. I am holding on to the right bannister, and Bill is descending slowly in front of me. The second to the last step—almost there.........I slip and fall and it's bad. I don't know if I slid because the steps were wet or if my knee buckled, but I went down twisting and bending back my entire left ankle and foot. We stayed for dinner despite my throbbing pain, which was eased by the glorious Tuscan red wine. We were there anyway, and I did not look forward to walking *up* the stairs. Always trying to be a "trooper." But why?

I spend the rest of November in recovery from the second fall. Taking baths in Epsom salts—the Italian version—and lying down with leg elevated with ice packs. But now I notice numbness in in both feet. I Google it: neuropathy. It persists.

I am off balance. I have eye floaters, and I have a sprained left ankle; and I refuse to go to an Italian hospital.

Chapter 7
HOME

December 2019

My currently undiagnosed situation has been going on for two years—but now I am in rough shape. The doc visits resume.

Bill takes me to Dr. Foot, our **podiatrist**, who x-rays both of my feet. Right foot reveals a former hairline fracture on right big toe that has healed. Left foot is not broken but ligament damage, still very painful after two and a half weeks, still swollen and bruised: top of foot, ankle, and outer side of ankle. He sends me for a nerve conduction survey with results sent to Dr. Rheumatologist. The following day, she calls and tells me I have to see her and get on medication immediately, as I have "polymyositis." This is my second diagnosis of the year.

Bill drives me to appointment, and we sit and listen. This is treatable with heavy duty drugs, but not curable. She prescribes methotrexate (don't drink alcohol) and continue with exercise. Like a giant baby, I am overwhelmed with emotion and cry. *How do I get something I never even heard of?*

I am dizzy from the medication, and we are supposed to leave for our usual Christmas trip to visit with our children and grandchildren. I tell my daughter we can't get to Chapel Hill, always our first stop. She says they will meet us in Boston, where our other family members live.

I feel desperate and completely out of it. I decide to call the **acupuncturist** I have gone to for several minor reasons over the past twenty years. I have two visits with Dr. Z, which balances me enough to resume some semblance of steadiness that enables me to be able to fly to Boston. I feel marginally better, but am still dizzy from methotrexate.

Our good friend in Sarasota, a physician, is upset to hear of my diagnosis. He recommends we see the country's expert on myositis. He knows him and makes a phone call. I have an appointment to see arguably the country's leading myositis specialist at National Institute of Health in Bethesda. He is also at Johns Hopkins.

Our doctor friend says, "Look, there are good doctors here in Sarasota if you don't have anything really wrong. If you do have a serious issue, get yourself to Johns Hopkins, Mayo Clinic, or Mass General."

Thurs, January 9, 2020

I am halfway through week five of methotrexate. Tuesday is the big event; we go to NIH in Bethesda, Maryland for the REAL answers. What exactly do I have, what type of myositis? Is it really polymyositis, or is it something else? My life is hanging on this, but I'm trying to act nonchalant. Anxiety is causing eye flashes; I try to stay calm. I've become almost a hermit. I don't want to go out or be with people. When I am in a crowded or noisy situation, I get eye flashes. Bill has been great and encouraging, but I don't know what he is really thinking. He tells me Bethesda NIH will be a quick fix.

Because I was warned that alcohol should be consumed at a minimum or not at all while taking the methotrexate, I have been abstaining from wine. In 34 days I have consumed three glasses of wine—one at a restaurant in Boston over Christmas while dining with Bill's sisters and their husbands, when I got hit in the head with a plate by a distracted waiter; one on New Year's Day with Bill when we went out alone and it was delicious; and one the first week of January, when our friend Brian made a lovely dinner for us and had an extravagant bottle of Montrachet. Usually it's two or three glasses per night, which equals 90 glasses in 30 days, which suddenly sounds like a lot of wine. Actually, it's a little less because we never drink on Sundays. But most of our friends drink this much or more.

I hope this regimen reduces the inflammation. Also cutting back on sugar, and how I love my chocolate. Last night I took a sip of wine and it tasted like poison. So generally I stick to sparkling water. Maybe I have toxic myositis. Remove the toxins and all will be well. But not Botox, I hope. Is that a body toxin?

So tomorrow I have the **chiropractor** and Saturday,

my fourth acupuncture. And then Bethesda for all the tests and the prognosis, which I hope is not "Get your papers in order." I really need to clean out my closets. I will follow Marie Kondo and throw out everything that doesn't bring me "joy." That's just about everything.

Sun, January 12, 2020

Trying to stay positive. I'll call it my "situation." And I'll get past it. Long boozy dinners sitting with friends in restaurants no longer work for me. I am bored and restless. I want to eat, get up, and go home. I just don't feel like any semblance of the former real *ME*. Or maybe *this* is the new real me.

I guess drinking calmed my social anxiety, because I no longer enjoy being in large groups. I'm not there yet. I can't hear and I can't seem to see. I feel out of sorts. Maybe I was always anxious. I learned I was funnier and more social when I drank. Did wine make me more interesting or did it make the other people seem so? Hoping for good answers and not a death sentence in Bethesda. My friend in Florence called her stage 4 colon cancer an "inconvenience" and rebounded. I hope a rebound is in order for me.

What The Answer Is

I have returned from my expert assessment at NIH in Bethesda. Official diagnosis following three days of tests, MRI, etc.: **Inclusion Body Myositis**—IBM for short: a chronic autoimmune disease. No medication works, so they advised not taking the prescribed methotrexate, which pretty much destroys your organs. Exercise in moderation to build muscle in my quadriceps. Bad news: There is no cure! Good news (seriously?): It's slow-moving. Mostly men get this disease. I have five brothers: maybe I was supposed to be the sixth male.

It took over two years, endless tests, and numerous doctor consults to get this diagnosis. This is the moment I will never forget. Feeling fucked! Feeling hysterical: WHY WHY WHY? It's not fair! Silent rants!!

Can I just say that I used to believe in cosmic credits? I thought that since I took care of my mother for eighteen years (the last five did me in) and have had other issues to deal with, like Bill's accident, I was covered—I paid my dues. No such luck!

You can use a challenge to awaken you, or you can allow it to pull you into even deeper sleep.

—Eckhart Tolle

Shoulda Coulda Woulda

I should have been aware of the warning signs that began in 2017, three years ago. My first annual physical where the doctor actually found a tiny health negative: low vitamin B12 with a suggestion to come in for a monthly injection. I had been experiencing extreme stress relating to my mother's care.

I begin to revisit if I made the right decisions. Should I have let her remain living in her own home? Would that have been considered elder abuse? She had numerous falls, but what if she'd fallen when I was out of the country and she had no one to call and take care of her? She did not want to move to assisted living; and she flatly refused to wear a "Help Me" button around her neck. Mercifully, the decision was removed from my hands when, leaving rehab after yet another fall, she was told by staff that unless she had 24-hour nursing care, they could not release her to live on her own; she needed more care and her demands were constant. I interviewed home health care professional services and presented her with the numbers, which far exceeded the cost of assisted living that "did not have to be forever"—and she chose B, the less expensive option.

Then there was the driving. "I have to die anyway" was her response. "But Mom, how about endangering the lives of others—what if you hit a car with a family? It might not be their time." She refused to listen to reason. My older brother called her the most stubborn person he'd ever met. In the end, that decision was taken from me as well, when she did hit a woman who, although not injured, claimed damage to her car. The state required an in-person test, the only part of which she passed was knowing the red sign with big letters STOP, so they took my 95 -year -old mother's license. All this caused additional anxiety—it was my life. I should have tried meditation or yoga. I was unable to detach with love. Yet I did not let this interfere with what I wanted to do, which was return to our beloved Florence for three months each fall and to Chapel Hill and Boston for Christmas to visit our children and growing grandchildren. She would journey to visit one of her four remaining sons for the holidays.

When home in Sarasota, I developed strategies and contingency plans. These included taking Bill with me to visit her at Assisted Living; she adored him and was always on her best behavior. Another relaxation technology included coming home, drinking too much wine, and downing handfuls of chocolate chips.

Then came the vitamin D deficiency followed by a urinary tract infection as soon as we hit Italian soil. I was neglecting myself and caring for others. My body was screaming for me to slow down and take a deep breath—drink less wine, drink more water, and learn relaxation techniques. Another UTI followed. I had to see an Italian doctor, who gave me some sort of powder to dissolve in 8 oz. of water. Somewhere along the way I should have noted that my immune system was in a downhill spiral. I was not dealing with the underlying problem. Emotions affect your health.

But health is about more than just overcoming illness. It's about maintaining a healthy lifestyle and living a holistic life—one in which stress and worry don't feature. Here's a thought: Surround yourself with people and things that bring you joy. I never addressed the deep-seated issue, which was that my mother and I never had the chemistry thing going. We were never buddies, and I remained terrified of her.

The five stages of grief (according to psychiatrist Elisabeth Kübler-Ross) **or pissed-off-ness** (according to me) **are:** denial, anger, bargaining, depression, and acceptance. I have covered all but number 5 because I am not accepting this. I have not had the biopsy, so maybe it's a misdiagnosis. I decide on partial transparency and I tell a couple of close friends.

Here's a good response from a real friend.

Thanks for letting me know, Susanna. I admit I have been worrying about you, and I guess this is relatively good news. Progression is slow; you don't need to take any drugs with horrible side effects; and you would be exercising anyway, which you mostly enjoy. Plus I'm sure it's a relief to know what's been going on and why you've been falling, having a hard time getting out of chairs, and so on.

But it still seems to me that you and Bill have been dished out more than your share of woes in the past year or two.

How are you feeling overall?

Want to have lunch when you are up to it? I know it's crazy-season, so whenever it works.

January 2020   Doctor Shaming—a New Trend

Dr. Neurologist follow-up. At the end of the month, I return to get an additional EMG, nerve conduction survey of my feet, on the recommendation of Dr. Expert at NIH. The cute young doctor proceeds to tell me off in no uncertain terms. He is not impressed that I went to the leading specialist in the country. He claims—as he bangs his fist on the desk—"This is MY disease." Dr. Expert said he was 99.9% sure it was IBM, but I should get a muscle biopsy (only at Hopkins) down the road.

To be clear, I did not go to the neurologist initially for myositis. I went for feeling off balance and headaches, as directed by my primary care doc. He sent me for a brain scan. I was scolded for canceling the appointment last June (I have a rational explanation), and he questioned the diagnosis of IBM since I did not have a biopsy. He sends me to PT at the hospital. Won't do an EMG unless I get two biopsies: one of thigh and another of upper arm.

Worrying is like paying a debt you don't owe.

—Mark Twain

New Year, New Physical Therapist

This turns out to be excellent, and I have a wonderful young therapist at Sarasota Memorial Hospital. She encourages me to "listen to your body" and follow a healthy diet of anti-inflammatory foods and controlled exercise. I now have a diagnosis, so she is referencing exercises specifically recommended for my disease of IBM. I am not happy that I have an incurable disease with no current treatment available. And then I run into an old friend, younger than me, who is in a wheelchair. Now I almost feel guilty, because her botched spinal surgery has left her paralyzed for life.

I see this all as a reminder that we should never take anything for granted. We should live in the moment as directed by Eckhart Tolle, extoling the power of now. I'll try harder. As Clint Eastwood said: "Tomorrow is promised to no one."

February 14, 2020

It is Valentine's Day, and Bill and I are at our art studio in downtown Sarasota. My doctor has sent a prescription for a handicapped car tag. The government office is nearby, so Bill suggests we go across the street and get it done. We walk over, and in fact they suggest a permanent handicapped license plate when they find out I am diagnosed with a chronic disease. I'm in a daze; Bill accepts the plate, pays the $40 fee, and we return to the studio. He gets a screwdriver and attaches the shiny new plate to the car. When I see it, I burst into tears. Bill suggests that the tiny wheelchair on the plate is cute and I will have my choice of prime parking spots. Since it is Valentine's Day, we drive to the Ritz for a lobster roll. There are no stairs to climb, and they valet my newly handicapped SUV.

Dr. Z acupuncture is scheduled every Wednesday. He is so positive and assures me that he can make me better. "I cure you." I believe him.

My doctor daughter suggests I should "talk to someone." I joke that I've read the book, *Maybe You Should Talk to Someone* by Lori Gottlieb, twice. "Seriously, Mom. Think about it. And maybe it would help to get a cane for stability." She doesn't believe in me or that I can get better.

I order a cane/walking stick from Amazon—for stability when Bill is not with me. It arrives the next day: Folding Cane, Derby Handle Walking Stick, Adjustable Collapsible Foldable Walking Cane for Men and Women, Blue Cyclone, Amazon recommended, $14.99

Am I giving in to the IBM? I have a terrible fear of falling, especially when I see stairs. I've got to stop Googling: too much information available on internet, and not always reliable. I am taking ginkgo biloba capsules for my eyes and doing eye exercises. It has not helped a bit, so fuck it. And I find a psychotherapist.

Chapter 8
MY NEW BEST FRIEND

Mon, March 2, 2020

I think that with all things in life, we need a best girlfriend to talk things over with—someone who makes us laugh and assures us that all will be fine. And if that fails—which in my case it did—then a psychotherapist is a good replacement.

I made an appointment with a therapist for a variety of reasons. First, I was trying to deal with my medical situation—to come to terms with and accept the uncertainty of my future. I did not want to burden friends and family with my day-to-day anxiety and questions pertaining to the cause or prognosis of the disease. They did not know the answers and often offered unsolicited and frankly stupid advice. I found an educated specialist in the chronic disease area who I hoped could calm down my increased anxiety and guide me through my uninvited and unwelcome journey. Hopefully she would reassure me that I could realistically expect improvement or at least to stabilize and convince me that ultimately all would be okay.

Rona turns out to be just what I need. A smart Jewish woman from New York, good sense of humor, understands the situation, and she specializes in patients with chronic diseases, which I apparently am. I save up my thoughts and fears all week to talk with her. Time to stand up and face the facts like a strong woman.

Rona does tell me, "Recovery of function is realistic" but I should "Focus on ability, not disability." I also need a sounding board to vent about my mother. Rona turns out to be more of a "go forward" therapist, as opposed to a psychoanalyst who mines the past to find out how I got here. Rona's response to my litany of complaints about my mother is, "She's dead, move forward. We cause our own suffering when we dwell on the thing that hurts us. Change the story! The past is unfixable—stay present and focused."

Of all the pictures of myself from my entire life—and there are many—there is one in particular that I love. It's not even a photo from my skinny modeling days and the many ads I appeared in over the years. It is the sepia-toned, professionally taken, First Communion photo of me at six years old, an age when I staged circuses and plays in my backyard with my best friend, of the same first name. I dig it out of the drawer, and I look into the sparkling innocent eyes of that little girl in the starched white organza dress and First Communion Headband Veil, full of hope and pride, and I say out loud, "We will take care of you and make you better—but start taking better care of yourself." I put the photo in a frame and place it on my desk so I can talk to her every day. We will walk her through this. I find the quote that I love from Shakespeare's *A Midsummer Night's Dream,* spoken by Helena in Act 3, Scene 2, referring to her friend Hermia, and I print it out and stick it behind the photo: **And Though She** Be **but Little She Is Fierce.**

March 2020.

And then the deadly coronavirus hits the world.

I don't have the energy to socialize anyway, and I am considered "high risk" because of my age and diagnosis. We are all wearing masks and hiding out.

Our friend in Boston was recently diagnosed with stage 4 lung cancer. She is fourteen years younger than me, never smoked, and is a superb athlete. So unfair. When we last met with Barb and her husband, she said with positivity, "I've got this! But I'm tired of filling out all the medical forms: Did I smoke? Nope. Do I drink? Yes. How much? Answer: Not enough." I laugh. "I know now that nobody actually reads those forms," she says.

May 2020

We are quarantining in the midst of Covid-19 when I spot a nasty looking small growth on my right lower leg. My dermatologist is closed, so I go to Bill's doctor for a biopsy, which comes back "Squamous." He says it must come out. I schedule MOHS surgery for the next week. It's very deep, and I have to return the following day for stitches. Lower leg heals slowly because of lack of blood flow: 27 stitches. Doctor doesn't believe in wearing a mask to prevent Covid. This makes me anxious. And so it goes. Trying to stay off leg. Hurts like hell. I have to quit PT so as not to put pressure on the wound.

Cancer surgery on leg set me back, as I am unable to walk a lot or ride stationary bike. I am feeling hopeless. I am letting Bill down, but he has been so encouraging and helpful and given no indication of me ruining his life. I am no longer the fun companion he signed up for 31 years ago when we met and married six months later—both for the second time. I was always up for anything, and we are great traveling companions and an extremely social couple. I'm known as an excellent party giver and entertainer. I cannot keep up the pace and wonder how this will affect him and us. The "fun couple" has been cut in half—reduced to one.

Sat, May 16, 2020 The Desperation Tango/ Strategies and Hysteria

In full panic mode I continue Googling and listening to every person who has an opinion and a suggestion. It seems everyone has at least one brilliant idea. This morning I woke to find this personalized email advertisement from Juve Tress—a hair-growth treatment. Have I mentioned my hair is falling out?

Good morning, Susan!

While you might be used to dumping your morning coffee grounds in the trash or sink, I know the perfect way to recycle them.

Believe it or not, these grainy leftovers do wonders for your hair and scalp.

Here are <u>three</u> reasons to add coffee grounds into your hair routine:

1. **They're packed with caffeine**
   This natural stimulant is known to block DHT, a hormone that shrivels your hair follicles and causes hair loss. . . . Caffeine also promotes blood flow in your scalp — a *must* for healthy, continuous hair growth.

2. **They're an antioxidant powerhouse**
   Coffee has a variety of antioxidants, including natural hair-savers called flavonoids . . . [that] can help improve your scalp's ability to fight off harmful free radicals, invasive molecules that make your hair look thin and dull. . . . Flavonoids also act like armor against breaking and splitting, giving your hair a healthier, more luscious quality.

3. **They're naturally exfoliating**
   The grainy texture of coffee grounds can help remove excess oil, dirt, skin cells, and product buildup from your scalp. . . . This can help unclog your pores, creating better conditions for healthy hair growth. . . . It also prevents your hair from looking flat and heavy...so you get an instant boost in volume.

Here's what you need:
- 3 tablespoons of coconut oil (olive oil works great too)
- 5 tablespoons of used coffee grounds (room temperature)

Here's what you do:
1. Mix your coconut oil (or olive oil) and coffee grounds together in a bowl.
2. Massage the mixture into your scalp for about 5 minutes.
3. Rinse the mixture out into your kitchen sink or somewhere it won't clog your plumbing (doing this in the shower might cause your drain to back up).
4. Wash and condition your hair as usual.

I recommend using the scrub about once a week.
Dr. Hal Weitzbuch, MD

P.S. If you have some scrub left over, massage it onto your face and neck. Caffeine is known to help reduce redness and puffiness, so it can really perk up your complexion.

I finish applying the treatment just as the doorbell rings, and I open it to a stunned Amazon delivery man—pungent coffee grinds dripping from my dirty-looking head and plastered around my eyes. I smile as I accept the box, never losing eye contact. I'm sure I was his topic of conversation that night at *happy hour* someplace! Did I end up with "movie star" volume and shine as promised? I don't think so, but maybe I increased blood flow!

Tues, June 2, 2020

I have been wearing an elasticized ankle support for seven months, since seeing Dr. Foot when we returned from Florence in November. I am still having difficulty walking, and my ankle is now very stiff.

I get an appointment for a second EMG from yet another neurologist. Being overly cautious, he would not allow Bill in with me, and in fact he insists I tighten the nose clip on my Covid mask. I tell him I fell in November and noticed numbness in my feet after that. He conducts the test and quickly confirms I have neuropathy in both feet. I ask what caused it. "Do you have diabetes?" "No." "Have you had chemo?" "No." "Do you drink alcohol?" "I drink a little wine with dinner. What can I do for it?" There must be a cure. "Nothing will cure it. Don't drink. Remember the old Western movies where the cowboys were drunk and stumbling around? They had neuropathy in their feet."

Driving home Bill says, "Seriously, he was comparing you to an old stumbling cowboy? Why didn't you tell him he was insulting and to go fuck himself."

I make an appointment with a foot and ankle M.D. orthopedic specialist. He looks at the x-rays. "Nothing is broken." He scans the nerve conduction study I hand him and says, "These numbers mean nothing to me: I'm a carpenter, not an electrician." There is nothing he can do—he's a surgeon. He tells me to go to PT for my ankle, so back to PT I go.

If you are depressed, you are living in the past; if you are anxious, you are living in the future; if you are at peace, you are living in the present.

—Lao Tzu

Chapter 9
BUILDING A TREATMENT TEAM

June 2020

Can I just say that I used to try for 10,000 steps a day on my Smart watch—easy in Florence, except for this year? Now I may manage around 5,000 a day, as we do shorter morning walks and we have not been out socializing for three months. I don't need to dress up for anything and I'm afraid to go anywhere but the grocery store alone. I wear a mask.

My face has a harried, drawn look and is too thin but thankfully the mask covers this. Bill thinks I should try to gain weight so my face will fill out.

I need to build muscle but must do it slowly so as not to create more inflammation.

I see Dr. Z for acupuncture and I find a neuromuscular massage therapist to help with my left ankle that I twisted badly on my second fall in Florence. I will see her this week for the first time.

No travel plans for sure, although Bill wants to go to

Boston at the end of July for our grandson's graduation from high school and stay for the month of August. I cannot think about that now, but I don't think I will give up my healing team and schedule here to go to Boston, despite the heat and our desire to see the grandchildren.

My vision is still blurry, which puts me off balance. Maybe I'm not used to wearing glasses. I keep switching from readers to distance spectacles. I told the ophthalmologist maybe I should try contact lenses. Just get up in the morning and put them in. But I still have the floaters that never left. I think most if not all of these issues that contributed to the falls came from anxiety. For usually extremely social people, I now find social situations create anxiety. I just broke down. Acupuncturist told me my current state is a result of too much stress. If I remove the stress and the toxins, why can't I get rid of the disease?

The plan going forward is exercise, acupuncture, rehab for ankle—massage and PT—and something for my eyes. I see a set of steps now and I freeze. I have to hold on to the railing with what Bill describes as "a death grip" and descend the old lady way—the sideways shuffle down the stairs, one step and bring the other foot, then next step and bring other foot, and hopefully make it to the bottom without my knee buckling. My mother was in great shape until age 94! It shouldn't be like this.

Wed, June 10, 2020

Return visit to acupuncturist. This time I bring my recent EMG study and explain about my left ankle and my feet neuropathy getting worse. He says he can fix it. When I leave after 25 minutes of needles sticking all over me, a cluster at my ankle and some in my head for anxiety, I feel notably better and more balanced.

Thurs, June 11, 2020

Today I go to my new massage therapist, who was described by my good friend as a "healer." Sarah released the fascia in my lower legs and massaged my feet extensively. She gave me some exercises to do. I feel I have a good team in place and am optimistic about some form of recovery or at least stabilization. If my ankle is better—currently it doesn't bend when I walk down stairs—I will not have such a fear of falling.

Fri, June 19, 2020

Our 31st anniversary was two days ago. We had a lovely day. Walk on beach in the morning, Bill working from home; I went for acupuncture and at the last minute we went out for an early dinner at Michael's on East "socially distanced" bar with Joe the piano player singing to us "It's a Wonderful World." I had to wear flat shoes. I still have a bandage on my MOHS surgery on my right leg, as it is still not closed up after six weeks post-op.

I try to take one day at a time. We walk daily still, but slower and not our usual distance. I get very tired at around 2:00 every day. Watching my wine intake carefully. Probably should quit altogether. Thinking of that. But I sure enjoy a glass of wine with dinner. How could that be bad for me?

Anniversary I had two. We did so much travel, and my "condition" is putting a damper on all of this. Sometimes I think, since I did not have the definitive muscle biopsy, maybe Dr. Expert made a mistake and I have something else that *is* treatable.

Psychotherapist suggests taking the focus off my illness. The redo of my latest book is done. I had to change the title. The publishing company was sold to Amazon and the software is different, creating a nightmare in the formatting. That was a lot of stress but it displaced my center of attention. **Forever Florence** is now live on Amazon.

After almost three months of Covid-19 precautions, my cleaning lady Gloria is back. I love her and need her.

My local team:

Bill, head coach

Dr. Z, acupuncture once a week

Psychotherapist bi-weekly

PT 2 times a week

Massage therapist once a week

Pilates, returning July 9, once a week

Sun, June 21, 2020

We were out three nights celebrating our anniversary. One night at a friend's house, two at restaurants. I am pooped. Friends invited us to socially distance in their yard yesterday, Saturday, for a cocktail. We'd already been out three times in a week—a Covid social record for us quarantiners. But we went anyway and stayed for two hours; now I am tired.

Mon, June 22, 2020

What a bad day. It has caught up with me. I can barely walk and am exhausted. I think I'll quit wine.

Found a book by accident—Kindle $3.99—about getting sober. Very entertaining yet poignant. Loved reading about this fortyish woman who gave up drinking. Maybe I should do it.

Thurs, June 25, 2020

Four alcohol-free days. I went to Sarah for a massage of legs and feet. Told her I had blurry vision. She said liver was directly related to eyesight. I come home and Google vision and eyesight and alcohol consumption. Make a note to ask acupuncturist next Wednesday if I have liver fire. Everything is connected. Imagine if I can get my eyes back without floaters? And my ankle and neuropathy better. Then I'd only have the IBM. I have a great team, possibly lacking a dietician who will inevitably advise against any wine, wheat, sugar, and dairy. Seems to be the trend. I will be a really boring person if I stop drinking, and Bill will say it's a deal breaker. He says I never drank that much, or he would have told me. My internal monologue in my head suggests maybe I should go for total sobriety—rid myself of all possible toxins.

Quitting my beloved wine completely would change a few things. Bill thinks I should have at least a glass of red wine every day. The exquisite and civilized habit of the aperitivo in Florence. The incredible Tuscan reds with dinner. I won't say forever. I'll say for now……one day at a time.

Tues, June 30, 2020

Nine days no wine. Lemon-flavored La Croix water is my new best friend. I think that I need to do everything possible to build back my immune system. I have to believe I can beat this. I will continue. It's easier to not drink when home, and we sure are home a lot now with Covid running rampant.

Psychotherapist Tuesday, now virtual. I'm explaining my stress came from dealing with my mother.

"She's dead, go forward," says Rona again.

Thurs, July 2, 2020

Massage: I open my eyes and see that Sarah is kneeling on the end of the table, hovering over me and stretching my legs over her head. She starts pounding my clavicle with a definite 1- -2-3 rhythm. This is my introduction to Thymus Tapping to reboot my immune system. I Google and find demonstrations on YouTube.

Meditation: I bring my body into healing and balance. One step at a time, one day at a time. Be strong—be grateful. Just do the next right thing and you will arrive.

Sun, July 5, 2020

Fourteen days alcohol free. Do I feel any different? No, but I will continue for 30 days, as this is also supposed to reboot the immune system. I will renew my body, mind, and spirit. Now doing Deepak Chopra 21-Day meditation. My mind wanders: *Did I put the wash in the dryer?*

DAY 1 Mantra: Ram [Ruhm]

English Essence: I activate healing in my body, mind, and emotions.

August 2020

The days run together as I religiously follow my weekly healing schedule. I have not been able to climb up the stone built -in steps to my master bath shower since we came home from Florence nine months ago. I am frail. I try getting quotes on making it handicapped-accessible, but every contractor just wants to gut the bathroom—a six-week project at great expense and not what we want. I can use the guest bathroom. Bill says, "Why not? We're not having any guests during Covid." I am too tired for guests.

Fri, Sept 11, 2020   The Myositis Association Virtual Conference

I sit at my desk and tune into The International Patient Virtual Myositis Conference over the weekend and check the agenda. I choose sessions where I think I will find some helpful and hopeful information, but as I watch and listen to the people at varying stages of the progression of the disease, unable to walk or swallow among other things, I experience fear and panic. I start to text Dr. Expert and tell him that I need to see him, but the bottom line is I need to get a biopsy for absolute verification of IBM. There is only one person who does it here in Sarasota, Dr. K Neurosurgeon. Dr. Expert prefers that he set it up at Johns Hopkins, which he trusts. I'm hoping to get into a drug trial. Expert finally agrees, quite reluctantly, that I can have it done here if the guy does quite a few of them and agrees to send the results as well as the slides to him. I'm thinking I'm better off at Hopkins. What do you think? I am wondering if fatigue is such a big part of this disease.

Sun, Sept 13, 2020

Fall is traditionally a time of renewal, as we look toward our vision of the future. No wonder it's my favorite time of year—despite the global pandemic and the disease that has been thrust upon me. I am hoping for a better future—have graduated from Physical Therapy and returned to Pilates. In my new reality I no longer think, *Why me?* The reality is: *Why the fuck not me?* I was chosen randomly, like so many other people with varying diseases. We are all struggling. Trying to stay in the moment. I am a Leo, I am a warrior. I stare at the photo on my desk of the six-year-old in her First Communion dress: "Never forget that you walked away from the monster marriage 48 years ago. You've got this!"

67

Life starts all over again when it gets crisp in the fall.

—F. Scott Fitzgerald, *The Great Gatsby*

Chapter 10
VITAMIN MANIA

As a senior, I face the risks from the prescribing cascade. I line up the supplements I have been accumulating and taking since January. It's out of control, and I am a person who does not like to swallow pills. Bill and I have always taken a daily Multi B vitamin (2) and Curcumin Q10 (2) and sometimes a Vitamin C. So that's five capsules a day.

My acupuncturist prescribed something called Bing de Ling twice a day, in addition to Lycii Chrysanthemum Teapills (6 twice a day) and 4 calcium with magnesium in hard-to-swallow large tablets (total 18). From my dermatologist I have Heliocare supplement and a Nicotinamide capsule (2) to help prevent further skin cancers. My massage therapist, in an effort to help, recommends and sells supplements: Nerve Support (2) and Nerve Repair (1) vitamins for my neuropathy. (Product description: Soothe Your Nerves! Nerve Control 911 acts as a safe, all-natural formula with results that rival Big Pharma's prescriptions and over-the-counter NSAIDs like ibuprofen, aspirin, naproxen, and acetaminophen.) She has also recommended Perfect Amino acids (5 daily) and something called InflammEnz (1), as well as LemonGrass essential oil for inflammation.

On Facebook I am drawn to heavily advertised Grass Fed Collagen Peptides promising glorious shiny hair, smooth skin, strong nails, and joint support. This also contains all the amino acids. *What harm can it do?* I order that as well. Then I have the vitamin D (1) and also clinical strength cranberry capsule because I had a UTI 2 years ago. This totals 36 supplements in addition to the collagen powder I put in my morning coffee.

At Bill's extremely strong urging, I make an appointment with my GP (virtual due to Covid) to review the list. I sit in front of my computer, iPhone propped up on Facetime, along with my bag of vitamins—some overlapping, probably causing toxicity. I hold each one up and tell her who prescribed it or if it was self -prescribed. We quickly run down the list from "Okay" to "Get rid of it," eliminating more than half.

Acupuncture, massage, and Pilates are not covered by Medicare. My treatment plan is expensive. But we are not traveling or going out during the pandemic, so I don't spend money on makeup, clothes, or restaurants—so it's probably a wash.

My Pilates instructor tells me that one of her clients has had success with his neuropathy with a treatment called Anodyne therapy. I make an appointment, but it is actually a PT place, and all I want is the light treatment for my feet.

Mon, September 21, 2020   Chasing the Cure

Monday, a new week—a new beginning. Bill and I drive over to the beach and have a glorious walk, me with the aid of one trekking pole. There's a break in the heat and humidity, which is sublime and leads to feelings of *I can conquer anything!*

I have not told Bill I am doing this because he would tell me I'm wasting my time with yet another "quack!" I'm going to surprise him with the miracle cure. So after breakfast I drive 30 minutes to a new Physical Therapy place that offers Anodyne therapy for neuropathy. My tingling and numb feet feel like they belong to someone else. They don't bend when I walk, and I'm clutching the ground with my unfeeling toes. By the time I arrive, I already know there is no way that I can drive this far two or three times a week because my days are already filled with all of my other appointments. I don't like the feel of the office, and everyone waiting is at least 300 pounds and has a cane. I don't want to be here—I'm in denial.

The therapist comes out, and according to Dr. Foot, who sent the prescription ahead, she presumes I am there to come to PT three times a week, followed by the heated red light Anodyne therapy. I am now a bit cranky and I tell her I'm not coming for PT, as I've been going since January (with a brief recess in beginning of Covid). I only want the machine therapy. She tells me it is all together in a package, yada yada yada. I feel exhausted. After much discussion, she tells me that insurance doesn't cover the treatment—they just throw it in with the PT package. They will let me come for just the Anodyne treatment at $25 per visit.

I ask if I can try it. So off come the shoes and socks, and out comes the black machine, which attaches to the outer sides of my lower legs and the bottom of my feet, and I sit for 30 minutes during the treatment. I pay and leave and trip in the parking lot—fortunately I do not fall. My feet feel worse. Not the panacea I expected, *and* you have to keep doing it; when you stop, it no longer helps.

But we need plants for the patio, and I am so close to Home Depot. I am in the plant department wearing my mask when I run into an old acquaintance who I haven't seen since January, but she knows that I have a health "situation" because there have been a number of things I've been invited to and I have bowed out, saying I have myositis and I don't feel well. She has a very loud voice: "Oh hi, I heard something was wrong with you." I say, "Yeah, I have this degenerative muscle issue, and my days have been spent with therapies, and not a lot of fun, social things." Her response is: "Well, I feel absolutely fabulous—I've never been better." I smile and reply, "Well, that's great!" And I convince myself that I meant it.

Anyway, that is my third activity of the day. On any given day I don't do well with any more than two activities.

I leave and go to Whole Foods—activity number four— Then I get home after 5 o'clock and actually make dinner.

Tues, September 22, 2020

So today I am non-functioning. Life goes on, one day at a time. *Piano, piano* (slowly, slowly), as they say in Italy. Stay in the moment, don't fret over the future. All we really have is today.

Fri, September 25, 2020

I think the most difficult part about this for me is my lack of energy. On the positive side, we are so lucky to live where we live and fortunate to be able to drive over to Lido Beach and walk on the sand and go in the beautiful warm Gulf water, and we try to do this every other day. Today we walked to the end of the beach and back, about a mile, and went in the water for half an hour, where I jump, swim, and walk backwards. The buoyancy allows me to do what on the ground I can only dream of doing. But now I am home and totally exhausted.

In my head a new deal is brewing—what if I can get into a drug study and I can stop the progression of this disease or turn it around; or what if miraculously the muscle biopsy shows that it isn't what we think it is and it's some other treatable disease? What can I make a deal about? What can I give up? What can I give back to society? This is only my second deal with God since I agreed to not do cool sculpting.

It's about attitude. I will stay positive and be grateful for today.

*I'll think about that tomorrow.
Tomorrow is another day.*

—Scarlett O'Hara in *Gone With the Wind*

Chapter 11
GRATITUDE

Still September 2020

Each morning when I awake it takes a few moments before I come to terms with my "new reality." I realize there are two ways I can deal with this: I can dwell on my condition or I can "stay in the moment," live each day, try to strengthen muscles, and pray for a cure. Practicing gratitude is also a wonderful way to improve how you feel instantly; to feel happier and more fulfilled. And I can be grateful for what I have. There are so many benefits of gratitude. It's wonderful for your body, mind, and spirit. I am so grateful I have Bill. I don't even mind his snoring now; it reminds me he is safely next to me sleeping. Today he walked me into the water with waves and undertow and uneven bottom of the Gulf. I could not have done it alone.

More than anything I'd like to have my energy back, more than being able to climb up a staircase without pulling myself or getting down a staircase without enormous fear of falling. My psychotherapist told me that "What you resist, persists." The anxiety will continue if I do not overcome it. Laugh more!

I gaze woefully into my shoe closet. The wedge shoes and boots that I wore only last year are a thing of the past, as I have worn nothing but sneakers for ten months. Remarkable how life can change so swiftly. In a recent *NY Times* story, a journalist interviewed Debbie Harry, the lead singer with Blondie and my age, about regrets. Her answer: "My only regret is that I can no longer wear high heels."

Speaking of regrets, I wish I had not stopped taking the prescribed HRT (hormone replacement therapy) that I had been taking post-menopause. My skin instantly aged about twenty years and I won't even discuss the beginnings of vaginal atrophy. It's so undignified. Once you've stopped taking hormones, there is no going back.

I try to follow Deepak Chopra and Eckhart Tolle and stay in the moment. I do try. I wake up in the morning and forget until I get out of bed, and then I recall I have Inclusion Body Myositis.

Preventing stress is key. I am trying not to worry about what is going to happen for Christmas. If I am unable to travel, will Bill go alone to Boston? Will I be here all alone, drowning in a pool of self-pity? Will I ever get back to Florence?

According to an Italian proverb, "If you have an easy-going and relaxed approach to life, you'll live more healthily and longer." And this is exactly the attitude I did not practice.

I always thought I was a survivor—actually more of a thriver. Life has thrown me a few curveballs, but I always rebounded and turned it around; lemons to lemonade—or often, Limoncello. The first of such being my first marriage, a penniless exit with my precious two- and three-year-old babies, wondering how I would ever survive; and yet I did. I stared down life's most terrifying challenge of raising two kids alone and succeeded. But this one—I don't know, maybe I'm too old. This is different; it's a physical issue that I can't seem to get on top of. Will it kill me? "No," the expert doctors told me; I won't die from IBM, but if I fall I could die, and falling is the big issue here. The progression to wheelchair is approximately fifteen years from onset, the expert tells me—if no major falls are involved. Since it took over two years for the correct diagnosis, I figure I am down to around twelve and a half years of trying to stay vertical. That's if I'm lucky.

I would like to emulate the words of the late RBG, Ruth Bader Ginsburg, when she said, "I'm going full-steam until I can't"—when she was ten years older than me and riddled with cancer. I'll believe the diagnosis, but not the prognosis.

Mon, September 28, 2020 A Down Day

If this is what the "senior" years are going to be like—I think I'd like to just take a pass!

At Hearing Institute for four hours of scheduled tests ordered by neurologist pre-Covid. Since Covid is probably never going away, I kept this appointment after rescheduling four times since March. So here I am.

I get a technician who has only been working here for three months. She is from the Bahamas. We do a balance test first. I can barely step up to the colorful, bright yellow box that looks like something in a preschool. But there are metal foot plates on the floor. So here's the deal: She outfits me with a harness like a paratrooper, I stand on the footprints, close my eyes, and the floor moves. I'm supposed to keep my arms at my sides and stand still. I open my eyes and notice that someone has punched through the right side of this playpen.

Now, I attempt to balance as the walls move—hands tight at my side. Cool! Close my eyes and stand still as the walls move, and now the floor jerks up: first a little, then medium, and the final all-the-way lift just about knocks me over. "Ahhh," I say to the non-communicative therapist, "I see why someone punched through the wall." I get a blank stare in response. Now the floor plates move back and forth, first a little, then medium, and you get the picture.

I'm exhausted as I follow her to the next room and the next test. I know this person is not a nurse. She doesn't tell me what the test is for, what to expect, or how long it will take. When I ask, she says, "You need to be quiet and stay still." Sounds blare in my right ear as a crushing sound resonates in the left. I say, "This loud noise can't possibly be good for my hearing." She admonishes me to be quiet.

Now comes my favorite part and third test—the booth. Again, she rams cone-shaped objects in both ears with no notice—then has to change them. I have small ears, she tells me. Noises screech in one ear as I strain to hear the word that comes in the other ear, which I am supposed to repeat. This goes on for quite a while, followed by me saying "yes" when I hear the different sounds. Ordeal over, I head to another room, where I pry out of her that this is for ear pressure. I really don't like this one. Feels like my brain is being sucked out, with my left and right ear fighting over who gets it.

The next room features a big chair where I am staring straight ahead at a green dot on the TV. She puts heavy goggles on me and asks about drugs. Have I taken sleeping pills or pain pills in the past 48 hours? No, but I was so nervous coming here that I took half an Ativan. What's it for? Anxiety. OOPS! Calls in supervisor. This is a no-go. Skip two tests and go to final. I am lying down when she suddenly starts to scrub my forehead. Me: "I have very sensitive skin; what are you scrubbing my face for? I have no makeup on." "This is a test to check for fluid. Again you need to be still and quiet"—as she turns up loud tapping noises in my ears, one at a time. "How long does it take?" "45 minutes". I am almost hysterical. She is now scrubbing my ears. "What are you doing?" "I need to place the electrodes."

My appointment with the doctor to discuss the findings is Wednesday. They are unable to reschedule the two missed balance tests for two weeks. I say fine, but I want a technician with a better bedside manner who has been there for a while. So I am to return for the remaining tests and see the doctor for the results.

The Power of Positivity and the Division of Lowered Expectations

My husband of 31 years is the most positive person I have ever met. In his mind, everything will *always* be okay—even when it's not! To him every day is a gift, delivering yet more wonderful opportunities for fun and creativity. In my case, he thinks there will be a cure for my chronic disease and I will be fine. Were it not for the Covid-19 pandemic, he would be making travel plans and thinking ahead as usual.

The second most positive person is Dr. Z, my acupuncturist. He is calm and reassuring and tells me the inflammation in my legs is gone and the disease has stopped progressing. Ever the cynic, I want proof. An MRI would show what's happening. The brain-to-body connection has just got to get jump-started. Dr. Z chats and smiles his infectious smile as he inserts the usual number of needles—somewhere between sixteen and twenty where needed. I instruct him to concentrate on the neuropathy in my feet. I can't understand his response because his Covid mask is thick, plus he chuckles and he has an accent. Perhaps I could eventually walk again in a low-heeled boot. Fortunately, clunky combat-looking boots are fashionable this year—not that anyone is going anyplace special. Combat boots and face masks: we look like a bunch of senior gang members. We all have choices in life. I choose to be with people like Bill and Dr. Z, who fill me full of hope and make me happy. "I fix you!" he says as he leaves me lying there in the darkened room, dreaming of recovery.

This journey is making me realize that I have to look at

what I have and not what I don't have. I have a wonderful husband, great friends and family, and an ideal place to live. My main goal is to stay focused and happy as I move forward through this *temporary* chapter of my life. Oh yeah, one more thing: Don't compare now to before; stay in the present; don't fear the future. Fear is the big killer here. And don't complain about flat, rubber-soled footwear as the only choice.

Psychotherapist: Stay fixated on the present. Past is unfixable: it's a recipe for misery.

It doesn't matter where the disease came from: finding a cause is not going to change anything. As the Harold Arlen/Johnny Mercer song says:

You got to ac-cent-tchu-ate the positive

E-lim-i-nate the negative

And latch on to the affirmative

Don't mess with Mister In-Between

You've got to spread joy up to the maximum

Bring gloom down to the minimum etc. etc. etc.

When Betty White was about to turn 99, she was interviewed for her *Parade* cover story in 2018. White revealed her secret to a long, happy, and healthful life: "Enjoy life," she said. "Accentuate the positive, not the negative. It sounds so trite, but a lot of people will pick out something to complain about, rather than say, 'Hey, that was great!' It's not hard to find great stuff if you look."

Betty also loves vodka and hot dogs, "probably in that order."

Never give up. And never, under any circumstances, face the facts.

—Ruth Gordon, American actress

Chapter 12
COVID BLUES

October 2020   Remembering PPE

In addition to my health and general feeling of being out-of-it, we are all dealing with the Covid pandemic. My kitchen has become a dumping ground for personal protective equipment—a mini-medical supply store. I have masks hanging on cabinet knobs and extra-large bottles of hand sanitizer and boxes of sterilized latex disposable gloves (no longer recommended by CDC) lined up on the counter, along with Clorox wipes that took five months to be back in stock. My life has become *Scary Movie # 3*. But I refuse to acknowledge any possible permanency of the pandemic situation by buying a new "Mask Friendly Hook System" as advertised in today's *Wall Street Journal*.

I also put masks and sanitizer in the car for extra precaution, as I live in terror of forgetting to grab my mask when I leave the house or—God forbid—not having my hand sanitizer with me at all times. I am considered "high risk."

Another benefit for us "seniors." Age and a compromised immune system make me a prime target for this nasty virus. Another reason to hurry up and put the business of my life in order so I don't burden my husband. I realize with amusement that if my obit says "She died at age 76," people will think, "Well, there she goes, she's had a full life—it was her time." No one will say, "She got robbed! (Of years) or "Pity—she was so young." We're all on the same path here. Better make the most of it.

Sun, October 4, 2020

I've been texting Dr. Expert at Hopkins and practically begging to come to Baltimore for a visit—anything that will get me closer to a clinical drug trial and a definitive diagnosis. He is at NIH and also Hopkins, but my understanding is that NIH is still closed. Is it dangerous during these times? Yes, we would have to fly and stay in a hotel, but we would be diligent and very cautious. I really want to get into a drug trial, and I really don't want my thigh cut open, but I really do want to know for sure what I am dealing with.

Rona says to stay busy and not dwell only on my "situation." "You're a writer: write something." Okay, how about these crazy Covid quarantine times? Or something like: *The Essential Quarantine Handbook.* Or ...

A Guide to Surviving the Pandemic of 2020

I'm on it: I'll make it humorous. This year has given us scores of new words, phrases, expressions and metaphors. Some are new to the popular vernacular, like social distancing, while others are newly relevant. Some are technical and others are medical jargon, but they could fill a small pocket guide. The sheer breadth of words that were popularized this year would be a good first chapter. The pandemic glossary: Social distancing, Super Spreader events, quarantine pods, Wuhan, cohort, contact tracing.

Zoom meetings, "out of an abundance of caution," panic shopping, curbside pickup, social bubbles.

There would be a chapter devoted to the Pandemic Wardrobe: masks, shields, protective clothing. The latest fashion in Hazmat Suits; face masks vs goggles and face Shields. A chapter on new ways of communicating and one on how to dress for Zoom meetings and Facetime.

I immediately lose interest. There is nothing funny about this pandemic. To make it seem so would be politically incorrect—at best. Too many people are dead and no end is in sight.

Mon, October 5, 2020   Vanity Returns

So what does one do between mandatory exercise like morning walks; riding the stationary bike for eight miles, 23 minutes; cleaning out closets and drawers; and keeping up with the more-often-than-not upsetting doctor appointments during the pandemic?

Outside, we wear masks and we have not been to restaurants for quite a while. So no need for makeup. My basic wardrobe currently consists of sweatpants and some form of Lululemon hoodie (with iPhone pocket) or half zip or long sleeve tee, and of course, the mandatory mask. The other day we were getting ready to attend a socially distanced birthday party of a good friend. My usual precision cut and highlighted hair of every three months is now long overdue for everything—screaming from the roots. It's been ten months since I've been to Vidal Sassoon salon in Boston. I dust off the mirror to see how I can "turn myself into a saleable commodity." (My younger brother used to tell me this is what I was doing if I wore any makeup, but that was at the beginning of the women's movement in the seventies He gave me two books, *Sisterhood is Powerful: An Anthology of Writings from the Women's Liberation Movement* and *The Feminine Mystique* by Betty Friedan, who years later, by sheer irony, rode with me by limousine as special guest to my book signing in Boston for my first book, *Real Women Send Flowers*. But that is a completely different story.

Anyway, I notice several circular brown spots on my otherwise dry and tired-looking face. I apply a light makeup and look closer but can't get past them. The next morning I call the plastic surgery center to inquire about options for facial discolorations.

Enthusiastic response: IPL helps treat these brown spots by selectively heating up the pigment (but leaving the surrounding tissue alone and unharmed), then lifting that heated, "damaged" area to the surface of the skin, where it is removed by the body's natural exfoliation process. A few quick zaps and four to ten days later—after the spots turn really nasty looking—they fall off. I'm in. I make an appointment, but I do not share this with Bill because he would tell me it is not worth risking my life for; I could get Covid. So I figure with any cosmetic procedure, he's on a need-to-know basis. The process is quick and cheap, and I know I'll feel a hell of a lot better when they are gone.

Dining In

"What's for dinner?" The perpetual question I am asked daily. For some reason, with all my cooking and baking, I am down fourteen pounds (probably muscle loss). "I've lost a stone." I always wanted to use the word *stone* in the weight category. The thing is, I own two scales. One is forty years old and digitally shows my happy weight, which is around four pounds lighter than the newer, accurate scale that Bill uses. "Why don't you throw out that old broken piece of shit?" he asks as I balance on it, tipping side to side until it stabilizes. "I prefer my weight on this one." But now I am recording my current weight on the two scales because I can finally tolerate seeing the number on the newer one. My hipbones are once again visible. Usually we go out four nights a week for restaurant dinners, drink wine, and eat relatively late. Now we eat healthy meals at home, and I am wine-free and thinner.

Wed, October 7, 2020

Weekly Wednesday with Dr. Z for acupuncture. He is convincing as he reiterates that there is no longer any inflammation and the IBM is stabilized: "No progression." I tell him my eyes bother me and I still have floaters. He says it is all connected to the IBM. Dr. Expert does not say this. When I relate this to Bill—and it all started around the same time—he says, "He's wrong. I'm beginning to wonder about this guy!"

Dr. Z is adamant about abstaining from any alcohol, even wine. So I do, and being home most of the time it is not difficult. The few socially distanced get-togethers have been easy, except the time outside at the restaurant with two good friends when I had eye flashes the entire night and had to pee but was hesitant to attempt the stairs alone in order to access the ladies' restroom. I think that when I drank wine, it took the edge off. Now the edge is back on and it has a name: Anxiety!

Mon, October 12, 2020

One week past IPL procedure, and sure enough the spots have disintegrated into what look like a few scattered coffee grinds where once the spots were. In a few days they should be only a memory. Now, if only I dare get close enough to another human being to brave a haircut. Bill, my most ardent admirer, inquires: "So, will you be getting your hair cut soon?" A wide, skunk-like streak of gray has appeared on the left top of my part, in addition to my hair being about a foot too long, kind of like how I wore it in my twenties when I was young and beautiful and my hair was thick and lustrous, which is no longer the case. On our morning walk, hubby proceeds to tells me a parable about a woman who lived near him in Massachusetts in the seventies. She was a psychiatric nurse married to a psychiatrist. An attractive brunette caught up in the women's movement who wanted to be liberated and decided to go "au naturel." She stopped cutting and coloring her hair and turned into a kinky-gray-haired hippie. Hmmm. I'm getting the message. I guess Bill does notice the gray streak. It looks like I won't be getting to my treasured haircutter and highlighter team at Sassoon in Boston this December. I make an appointment with a local.

Lisa Sanders, M.D. is a contributing writer for the Sunday *New York Times Magazine*. Her column is called "Diagnosis": solving the most baffling medical mysteries. I always look forward to reading it. I am thinking of pitching her the story of my ordeal: "The Road to Hell is Paved with Diagnoses." But she only takes cases that have been solved, and I know she would say a biopsy is needed for definitive diagnosis. Perhaps post-biopsy. Because then I will truly know. But I wait and wait for an appointment at Hopkins. Patience is not my strong suit.

Tues, October 13, 2020

I am forever seeing articles about famous people, actors or athletes, getting struck with a terrible disease. They fight and they say, "I won't let this disease stop me" or "I won't let this disease define me." "I have to learn to live with the disease and make the most of every day." Sounds good. I'm going to go with that flow.

Feeling inspired, we invite new neighbors over for "a drink." I go to the gourmet grocery and buy lovely paté, cheese, crackers, and hors d'oeuvres. I set up small appetizer plates and forks, napkins, ice in the crystal bucket, flowers on the table. House is perfect, and they arrive at six, at which point I am already exhausted. The most diffi-cult thing about autoimmune diseases is that others often can't see any symptoms so no one can really understand what I am going through. If I talk about it, it sounds as if I'm complaining, so generally I say nothing. We sit and chat, and by 7:30 I want them to leave, but Bill, always the entertaining host, is regaling them with stories. I'm drinking sparkling water with lime, which looks like the vodka tonic they are drinking. They switch to red wine. It's after eight when the man suggests it's time to go home and have dinner. I stand up, but Bill says, "No, stay and finish the wine." I want to shoot him. When they finally leave, I pour myself a full glass of red wine, cook and eat a hamburger, pour another glass of wine, and open a box of chocolate chip cookies, and devour half the box. This is not in line with reducing stress or sticking with a diet of anti-inflammatory foods.

I awake cranky the next morning following a much interrupted night's sleep. Something has to change.

Wed, October 14, 2020

My health needs to be the priority this year. Rona-thera-pist tells me, "You've got a double whammy going on: the pandemic and your medical situation."

Bill and I need to have an open discussion about Christ-mas now and get it out of the way. We have to stay home for the holidays, just like we did in 2016 when he was recovering from his accident, also for health reasons—this time mine. I am too vulnerable to Covid for rides in planes, boats, trains, and Uber cars. Sometimes men (penis brains) don't understand the obvious. And I can't entertain right now. I just can't do it.

Dr. Z pats my head and tells me to relax. "I cure you." When I leave the acupuncture office, I always feel less anxious and generally more stable. My knees have stopped feeling wobbly.

Dancing Knees

Sarah, my wonderful massage therapist, is also a yoga instructor. She gives me tips for stretching and strengthening by demonstrating a yoga pose. Today she tells me to do 100 strengthening knee flexes a day on each knee. This becomes part of my daily regimen.

Thurs, October 15, 2020

This is the day I return to the hearing and balance Institute for the final two tests that I could not complete two weeks ago. Today I have the good fortune of a lovely, gentle man who has been doing his job here for 31 years. He carefully explains what the tests will include. For the first test, I am sitting in an uncomfortably upright chair wearing 50-pound goggles, a required Covid mask covering my nose and mouth. I have to keep my eyes open as the chair moves and follow dots on a screen in front of me. The therapist is asking me the names of countries that begin with different letters, then vegetables, followed by men's names: "Can you tell me a man's name that begins with the letter O?" It is starting to feel more like a cognitive test. This lasts 30 minutes. There are cameras in the goggles (explaining the heaviness) that record my reactions.

We go to another room for the second and final 45-minute test, where I am instructed to lie down on a padded examination table. Once again I am fitted with heavy goggles which are darkened now, nose and mouth still covered with mask for Covid. First, hot air is pumped into each ear for one minute each side, and then the same with cold air. I am slow-breathing and counting backward: *You can do this—mind over matter*. I know I did not ace this test. Once again he is saying, "Name an animal that begins with letter J, now with letter K," and so on. The 50-pound goggles come off, and the room is swirling about me. I am clutching at the sides of the table, hoping I won't fall off. "Do you feel dizzy?" *Who wouldn't?* Mercifully, he directs me to look at three red X's on the ceiling. I stare and steady myself. I would not wish this on even my most hated enemy. Okay, maybe I would!

I'm wondering if I should tell him that I have a noise in my left ear—a sort of swooshing, dull thumping sound with a regular beat—almost like a loud pulse, always the same. But he will ask how long it has been there, and my answer would be, "I don't know." I usually hear it when I am in bed at night reading, and I always thought it to be the noise of the ceiling fan going around. Until I looked up last week and saw that Bill had turned the fan off.

Next week I will bring Bill (whether they like it or not—new Covid rule, patients only) to meet with the doctor for the answers: 1) What is wrong with my head, making me dizzy and unstable most of the time? And 2) What can they do about it? Hey, maybe a drug can fix the problem.

A Glimmer of Hope

Today, in complete desperation, I email Dr. Expert at Hopkins:

Dear Dr. E,

I wanted to touch base with you regarding my condition as well as a personal visit with you.

Since my meeting with you in January of 2020 and my diagnosis of IBM, I've been doing the strengthening exercises as you recommended; walking, stationary bike, Pilates, and those given to me by Physical Therapy.

I do not feel like I am getting any better; in fact, I feel like my knees and hip joints are getting weaker. So I am frustrated. I would like to know if you recommend I see someone locally in Sarasota who can possibly monitor my condition before I get together with you again. If so, would that be a rheumatologist or a neurologist?

I look forward to hearing from you.

All best,

One hour passes and he responds that he is sorry to hear my condition is worsening.

Unfortunately, this is what we would expect in those with IBM because the disease is progressive and has no known effective treatments. If you would like someone to monitor your condition, I would recommend that you see a local neurologist.

Dear Dr. E,
Thank you for your response.
I forgot to ask if there is now a clinical trial for IBM
I might be eligible for either now or in the future.

This doctor is direct and gets things done. He gets back to me within the hour. He tells me, "I heard through the grapevine that there will probably be a new IBM trial at Hopkins (and other centers in Europe and Australia) in the next year. If you are interested, may be worth seeing Dr. Tom Lloyd at Hopkins, who would be leading the Hopkins trial." I read it out loud to Bill, choking up. "Great, tell them we'll take Italy," he says. "See? I told you everything was going to be fine."

The Goodest Husband

When our now teenage granddaughter was about three years old and wanted us to take her to the store or for ice cream, she would try to persuade us by saying, "I'll be the *goodest!*"

Bill and I have been married for 31 years and we've been through a great deal together. An unlikely match at first, we have morphed into what he calls *one person*. He truly is the goodest and best friend and husband. Is this what couples mean when one of them says, "my better half" or "my other half"? We are in this together, which makes me fight even harder to get past my unexpected and unwelcome "situation."

Mon, October 19, 2020

A restful weekend. A new week filled with new information, and a haircut and highlights on the horizon.

My anxiety issues continue. In following up with the advice of Dr. Expert, I will try to find a local neurologist who can monitor my condition and understand that I am in the care of an expert. A doctor whose ego doesn't feel threatened by this. The same recommended name comes up three times, and I call his office. This neurologist has recently closed his successful neurology practice and has changed over entirely to a medical marijuana practice. Hmmm. This could work. Grandma Susan gets stoned!

Wed, October 21, 2020

Yesterday, in celebration of life, I did 24 minutes on the stationary bike, and Bill and I headed out to play nine holes of golf. It was a gorgeous day on the course, so just riding in the cart with my husband was joyful.

Today we go for results of eight hearing and balance tests. Bill tells me the doctor will tell me I need hearing aids. I'm okay if this is all. But I do think there will be an inner ear issue that shows up, and I hope he can give me a drug to help with my feeling generally out-of-it. If not, it must be anxiety, and I will pursue the now trendy CBD route.

Bill and I sit in the waiting room, and I am reading a poster on the wall about Meniere's disease. *I probably have this,* I'm thinking. The nurse comes and leads us into the examining room. *There never seems to be any resolution despite numerous tests.*

Doctor enters, nods at Bill and me, pulls up a seat across the room, and starts to check my test results on his computer.

"Minor hearing loss in left ear." *No shit!* "Right ear is a little worse, nothing too bad. Something is not getting to the brain. Could be a minor blockage or closed tube." He would recommend an MRI. Okay, I can do that. "Could be from a trauma to the head." (Like falling off a train and cracking my head on concrete pavement. Oh yeah, there was also the thick, glass one-liter bottle of Italian olive oil that fell off the shelf and onto my head.) I say nothing.

We progress to my three hours of balance tests: the playhouse with the moving walls and moving metal steps on the floor. Doctor intensely studying the notes. *Is this where he's going to tell me I have a brain tumor?* He looks up from the computer and smiles: "You passed all the balance tests...'with flying colors.'"

Wow. This all seems pretty good until I hear him say to the nurse, "Book an MRI with and without contrast." Hmm. I already know I don't want to be injected with dye. "I don't want contrast," I say. He, of course, responds that the only way he can tell if there is a tumor or any blockage is with contrast.

Return home, Google MRI with Contrast: **Contrast** is invaluable when imaging tumors in major body organs like your **brain** or in your central nervous system. **MRI** dye can help doctors detect the tumors, identify if they're malignant or benign, and determine the growth stage they are in. Do I proceed?

I throw the question out to my medical Board of Directors:

Friend Dr. Paul: *You need to get the test done with both. It will probably come back nothing but get it done. Having without contrast will not be helpful.*

Son-in-Law Dr. Dave: *You need that test the way they are ordering it. Good that the balance tests all check out!*

Dr. Daughter: *Hi Mom—Glad things were ok so far. Not useful to get the MRI unless you get it as recommended—contrast is needed.*

RN *Friend in question:* (She's already got the diagnosis?)
Great news! Is this your first MRI with or without contrast?
I think you may have had a linear skull fracture...
MRI will be definitive.

I have never had any procedure with dye. The idea of

shooting dye into my veins that will light up an issue in my head is frightening. But I'll gather my wits about me and do it. UGH!

In the meantime, today, following Pilates, I will go for a haircut and highlights, if for no other reason than to stop Bill from looking wistfully at my graying stringy locks. "Just get it cleaned up a little," he said most recently. "And cover the gray on the top." The bonus is—I know it will make me feel better.

Sat, October 24, 2020 It's All About Relationships/How to Unfriend Your Oldest Friend

I have not figured out the *how* but the *why* is because, for the past year, every time I talk to my oldest friend, I have a negative reaction, so it's self-preservation at this point. Yesterday, she called for advice on an upcoming family holiday. We talked for a bit, and then she asked almost in passing, "So how's it going?"

I explained that I'd had a good week, had just gotten a great haircut and color, and was in line for a clinical drug study at Johns Hopkins in an effort to find a treatment for my IBM disease.

"Oh good, you're finally doing something for science. Before my friend died, he donated his corneas and joined a drug study."

Another jaw-drop moment. *What the fuck is she talking about?* I take a deep breath and let it out slowly. "I'm not doing it for science. I am doing my best to stave off a wheelchair as my next means of transportation. I'm trying to stay vertical."

"Oh, ha ha, I love that, trying to stay vertical! I think I'll use that line."

Tonight I am restless and have a bad night's sleep.

Psychotherapist: She's not your friend. How many of these stories do you have to tell me?

Okay, she doesn't lift me up; she is no longer the "Wind Beneath my Wings." Perhaps she never was. My mother never liked her. "She's a user."

I have a shocking capacity for naïveté or maybe I've just always been a lousy judge of character, but I've ignored her lies and forgiven her transgressions by accepting any excuses—since grammar school. It's been said to never trust a dog that bites you because he will do it again. I've had to be bitten over and over before I come to the stark realization that she is not my friend. Mentally I start rationalizing by making lists of wrongs. There were episodes where I did not talk to her for a year at a time but eventually I would give in and forgive. I am not looking for sympathy, but perhaps a bit of empathy from an old friend who happens to be a health care professional.

From Oprah's "What I Know for Sure" *column interview with* Maya Angelou.

Oprah Winfrey says many of the most important things she knows for sure were gleaned from Maya Angelou:

"When people show you—or tell you—who they are, believe them the first time" is my all-time favorite.

("Baby," she once chided me, "they show you and show you, and you still don't believe what you see! Why does it take you 29 times?" That conversation was life-changing for me.)

My oldest friend relationship had come to an end. My life is in jeopardy. It's difficult to defriend someone with whom you have a long history—she's part of my identity and I loved her. We were the co-keepers of each other's memories. I'll break up over e-mail. I'm such a chicken.

Chapter 13
LOSSES

Sun, November 1, 2020

My good friend died from Covid on Thursday after four weeks on a ventilator. She was 69. The funeral is this week. Our life goes on: I'm lucky. I agreed to have the MRI with contrast this week. I'll have to be in a closed tube with crashing and banging for 45 minutes as they inject dye into my veins. Don't know if I want them to find something or not. But I'm better off than my recently deceased friend.

Wed, November 4, 2020

They had an open casket, and her husband and daughter were tragically and sadly trying to process the unexpected death and their loss. So were Bill and I. "No open casket when I die," I say as we get into the car to drive home.

Fri, November 6, 2020

The day of the dreaded brain MRI with contrast. *Mind*

over matter, mind over matter, mind over matter. I will get through this. I should have brought my mother's rosary beads, but leaning toward science, I took an Ativan. Should have taken two.

As I feared, it was horrible—complete with cage locked over my face and unable to move. I was so nervous before arrival that I didn't have a chance to be worried about the results, which I won't find out for three weeks unless the doctor has a cancellation prior to that time.

Mon, November 16, 2020

In talking to my daughter this past weekend, I mentioned that I am nervous about waiting so long for the results of the brain scan. I also said that I had called to express this, and the practice did not return my call. "Mom, call first thing Monday and tell them that it is bordering on malpractice that they have not given you the results of the MRI." I repeated this to my doctor friend here, who has always been so helpful. He said he respectfully suggests that I not do this, or there would be a good chance I would be fired as a patient.

But I do call, and once again express my anxiety at Day 10 post-MRI, saying the thoughts of waiting another three weeks were causing me a great deal of stress—which in turn aggravates my immune disorder. I am very assertive with the office and firmly plead for a callback. After an hour the phone rings with an offer of an appointment in three days, which I graciously accept. It's a lot of work trying to stay alive, chewing, and vertical.

Tues, November 17, 2020

After months of an ongoing toothache with the dentist telling me nothing shows in x-rays, I get a referral to the endodontist, but not before regular dentist on whom I have spent a small fortune tells me, "It may be a raging infection and you may lose the tooth." I say, "I really do not want to hear this." All this and a bill of $227, including a charge for personal Protective Equipment—I guess theirs, as I wore my own mask.

After one missed appointment due to hurricane flooding and high winds, I arrive the following week to meet my tooth fate. The good news is the bone is fine and there is no "raging infection." The bad news is that the throbbing Bicuspid (two canals) is in dire need of a root canal. The charge for CBCT scan and consult: $275. I try to make friends, telling the endodontist that I was pals with the former owner of the practice. (We were not exactly friends but I liked him.) It works and he agrees to fit me in at 4:30 the same day. Good news, I think. Bad news: $1,620 and a numb and swollen left side of my face. More good news: the dutiful and loving husband drove me for the procedure and is waiting to take me out to dinner with a glass of wine. The wine drools out of the numb left lip. $2,122 for one tooth that still requires a restoration.

Thurs, November 19, 2020

MRI results: No tumor. No evidence of internal auditory canal mass or labyrinthitis to explain patient's symptoms. What a relief. *So it's all in my head!*

"Where do you want your first cocktail?" Bill asks as we leave doctor's office.

Fri, November 20, 2020   Medical Marijuana

The noted and respected neurologist, now turned "Neurology of Cannabis" physician, calls himself "Dr. Tom." Apparently his last name is no longer essential to his new profession. We meet for the first and possibly only time, via virtual phone call. First of all, he tells me that the meeting with him, which will yield a prescription, will cost me $250. "Do you have a credit card ready?" Wow, that was a ho-hum crasher. Oddly, he was my choice for local neurologist with excellent credentials in neurology, as well as neuromuscular disease, and Medicare would have paid for the visit. But cannabis is cash!

Once past the finances, he asks what my issues are and if I have a problem getting to sleep at night. I do not. "How about waking up and not being able to get back to sleep?" Nope. I seem to have chronic anxiety! He doesn't seem interested in my diagnosis or why I experience anxiety. Dr. Tom recommends a vaping pen and holds up a sign with numbers so I will know what to ask for. I tell him I do not want to inhale anything, but he insists that it is perfectly safe: "Look, this is my wife's vaping pen. She uses it every night." *Does he love his wife?*

Tues, November 24, 2020   The Golf

Bill and I try to play nine holes of golf together every Tuesday afternoon. "Write it down like it's a weekly appointment, so you don't schedule something else," Bill says.

He is a great golfer who has been playing since college; I am a beginning golfer. What I enjoy most is riding around in the golf cart with him on a beautiful sunny day. The bonus is when I can hit the ball a decent distance and in the right direction. We always have fun. Today I play the first two holes before becoming overwhelmed with exhaustion. So frustrating as I sit out the third hole. No matter what I do or how much I rest, I am always tired.

Oliver Sacks, in his book *Gratitude,* describes a "sense of health and energy" that started to decline following his terminal diagnosis of metastatic liver cancer: "I have a pervasive tiredness, with sudden exhaustion if I overdo things." I can relate.

The Last Dinner Party

We owed, Bill urged, and I felt I was capable of having dear friends for a casual dinner. The only problem is, I never do parties in a casual manner. I decorated the entire house and put up the Christmas tree with the help of my design friend-elf, Steve. I put a lot of effort into buying, preparing, and cooking the dinner, setting a beautiful table, and making sure the house is immaculate and festive, in my goal of emulating hostess guru Martha Stewart. I simply can't help myself. This has always been something I loved doing, but now I am challenged by chronic exhaustion. I do what I can ahead of time—prepare food, set table, fresh flowers, house perfect—and by 5 o'clock I am crashing and think I can't get through it. Bill arrives to find his wife mid-nervous-breakdown with guests arriving in one hour. "What can I do to help?" And so miraculously, I rebound with the aid of half an Ativan and Bill's help, and we pull off a lovely evening. They leave at 11, we clean up the dishes, and go to bed. "I can't do it anymore," I say. Bill holds my hand as we fall into a deep sleep.

I tell Rona the story and she listens intently: I say, "If you don't go, you don't owe." She says, "Can I have that line?" Of course.

Tues, December 8, 2020
Where There's Dope, There's Hope!

The Medical Marijuana card has been processed. I can now legally purchase medical cannabis in the state of Florida—proving it's never too late to take up a drug habit. I have a list of stores and Google the one closest to me.

Located in a small shopping plaza, next to a dentist office, I find a discrete, pristine-looking white sign with a leaf and the name of the company: Greenleaf. There is no mention of what lies within. It's a cool December day as I pull open the heavy glass door and enter a small lobby with a reception desk. It looks more like a medical office than a drug outlet, and for a moment I think I've come in the wrong door until I spot the male receptionist sporting a streak of purple in his otherwise brunette hair, in addition to many jangling bracelets on both wrists.

After I sign in and hand over my new card and my driver's license, a young, attractive, heavily tattooed woman greets me and leads me to the back larger room. Smiling, she goes behind the counter: "I'm Tess; meet me at the fourth computer." I remain focused on her nose ring which looks eerily like the ones animals wear. I Google as I wait: A **nose ring** is a **ring** made of metal designed to be installed through the nasal septum of pigs (to prevent them from rooting) as well as domestic cattle, usually bulls.

I wonder if Tess's parents are happy with her appearance. She is a trim and attractive young woman and sounds intelligent as she explains the products. "Do you want to get high?" *Do I look like I would?* I am past wanting anything other than to be able to function and stay vertical. I tell her I have anxiety and I don't want to get high, vape anything, overeat, gain weight, or act stupid.

"Got it!" She turns behind her, opening white cabinet doors and pulling out drawers.She presents me with my options, laying them on the counter: tinctures, fast-acting Nano chews, even a balm to rub on pain areas. Today as a first customer, I get 50% off all products. Whoopee!

The newly crowned queen of cannabis leaves with confidence and her purchases.

I try the tincture marked PM and stay awake most of the night. I swear it energized me.

The next day I cut a Nano chew—the size of a nickel—into quarters. When I will be home and not driving, at 3pm, I take one piece. Five o'clock—nada. Nothing at all. I feel exactly the same.

I tell my doctor pal, who has experimented himself: "Start low and go slow," he says. "Try more tomorrow and see what happens."

No

It's taken me all my life, but I have finally found and believe in the power of no—with the help of therapist Rona. Saying "no" means I'm not doing things I don't want to do, so it eliminates the resentment. After all, for most toddlers, one of their first words is "no." They know what they don't want and they verbalize it. We get older and we learn to be more tactful.

We talked about obsessing about things that might happen in the future, including numerous social episodes—this creates anxiety. Rona relates a parable.

Here's the short version: A man's car breaks down on a lonely road. He has no tools to take off the wheel and change the tire. He sees a house in the distance and wonders if it would be okay to knock on the door—at such a late hour—to borrow a wrench. He is so nervous that the entire walk to the house he pictures a man woken from bed, yelling at him that NO he doesn't have a wrench and how dare he knock on the door, etc. He is so worked up that by the time he gets to the front door and rings the bell, a kindly old man answers and says, "Hello, how may I be of help?" The guy shouts at the old man, "You can take your fucking wrench and stick it up your ass."

Setback Saturday

I decided that I could do a weekend cocktail party for six people during the holiday season. No dinner, so this would be easy—good friends, very casual. Of course nothing with me is really very casual, but I had plenty of time to make some hors d'oeuvres and tidy up the house, and then I went to take a shower after I rode the exercise bike for 20 minutes. I am feeling a little tired as I get into the shower, and I drop my shampoo on the floor and try to pick it up. This is an exercise I've been practicing almost daily. I try to squat down as far as I can, put one hand on my thigh for support, and lean over to pick up whatever I've dropped.

Today as I stepped into the shower it didn't work. I couldn't reach it and somehow lost my balance and fell. I don't want to tell Bill this because he'll say cancel the party, and I really don't want to do that because now all the food is made and the house looks so festive. In some ways, he is so much smarter than me. I am just too stubborn. So here it is, 3 o'clock. I take two Advil and lie in bed with an ice pack on my foot. Mostly I'm mad at myself: *How the fuck did I let this happen?* I had a sound night's sleep and was feeling pretty good, but I think I pushed myself on the bike. This was an accident and accidents happen and my toe is throbbing and I hope it isn't broken. When I fall, I never do it gracefully; I always do a lot of damage.

I guess this is my last cocktail party. I'm really just not me anymore. I'm not up to that much, and I was so optimistic and so hopeful just yesterday. Now, I just want to get through tonight, knowing it will be the end of my entertaining. I rub the cannabis cream all over my foot, hoping it will help.

Tues, December 15, 2020

Yesterday I emailed the nurse at NIH and Hopkins. I explained my frustration at trying to get into a drug trial. I've been forgotten because of Covid. Somehow, through a couple of chatty emails, I feel a connection. She says we will double-team them and get something going. Today, miraculously, I get a message that his first appointment is in February or March 2021. I'm happy. An hour passes, and I receive an email asking if I could be available this Friday, in two days, for a 1pm teleconference. I'm ecstatic.

Wed, December 16, 2020
The Body Whisperer

I wonder if I have learned my lesson: "Listen to your body." I get so tired after walking on the beach. Today I also have acupuncture. I ask Dr. Z about medical marijuana and he is adamantly against it. He tells me it disrupts the digestive tract. Some people vomit from it. He goes on to tell me that the cows who live in close proximity to the fields where cannabis grows in China are sickly. Well, I was just asking, because it didn't really do what I expected. I'm feeling kind of down.

My unplanned for and unexpected health challenges have been an immensely difficult journey. But it has been a learning experience, which in itself is a gift. It allows me to take nothing, even the coming day, for granted. It also makes me feel grateful for what I have. Today I am grateful that I can walk (albeit slowly) and I can drive. That's a lot to be thankful for.

Fri, December 18, 2020
Light at the End of the Tunnel

The result of my frustrated and persistent email is a 40-minute teleconference with Dr. Lloyd, who will be starting a clinical trial for Sirolimus in 2021. Naturally Covid has knocked most things back, and this is no exception. He is waiting for the vaccine and would like to see me at Hopkins after I have been inoculated—possibly in May. He said that after reading Dr. Expert's notes, he concurs that he is 95% sure I have IBM, but I would need a muscle biopsy to be part of the drug trial. So I see all this as some form of "light at the end of the tunnel," though not the panacea I had wished for. It's not as if I'll be back to skipping or wearing high heels, but if it keeps me out of a wheelchair, I'll take it. No prejudice against people in wheelchairs intended. I just don't want to be a member of the club prematurely.

Thurs, December 24, 2020
Never a Real Athlete

For as long as I can remember in my adult years, I exercised. When my two children were toddlers, I would lie on the living room floor as they played nearby and follow the home exercises illustrated page by page from *Miss Craig's 21-Day Shape-Up Program*. Marjorie Craig was one of the pioneers of women's fitness. This book taught you how to improve your posture, alignment, and flexibility, and strengthen your core through a series of safe, easy-to-understand, fun, and interesting home exercises. The only equipment you needed was 3 lb. ankle weights and 3 lb. barbells.

I never fully embraced the next level of the glossy, overwhelming Jane Fonda's workout video—and frankly I found some of her exercises too difficult to emulate. But that was the seventies, and I was newly divorced, the sole breadwinner, and had to stay in shape, or I would not work in my profession of photographic model and TV commercial actor with no speaking lines. I just had to show up and look good. This also meant I could not gain weight, so I was always careful with my food choices.

As time passed, it seemed I always walked quite a bit, occasionally tried to run—but feared something (like an old IUD) was going to dislodge and fall out. I rode a bicycle on the streets of Cambridge, where I lived, skied occasionally when I could afford it, and went to the gym when I could. I even did a stint of adult ballet lessons. I was never what you would call an athlete, but I was physically fit enough. Nothing really held me back.

In my early childhood and formative years, to my best recollection, we did not have any type of formal exercise. My parochial grammar school in Bergen County, St. Peter's, was crammed with too many students (60 per class) and not enough nuns to keep it together. We were allowed outside on the "playground"/parking lot to stand and talk. (Some of us tried to sneak to the woods behind the buildings and smoke cigarettes.) And although there was a gym, it seemed to be used for 7th and 8th grade dances only. I have no recollection of any form of exercise taking place there.

The same could be said for my high school. There were sports teams for the boys, of course: basketball, football, track, and baseball. For the girls, the only form of sport was rooting for the boys in the form of cheerleading—jumping up and down in short skirts and screaming "Go Team Go." Growing up in the suburbs, we rode bikes and roller skated. That was pretty much it. Figure it out for yourself. Go out and play and don't come in until you are called for dinner. We walked everywhere. One car shared by our family with six children. Don't even ask for a ride! Now a girl can't graduate from high school without Physical Ed. Our grandchildren are given their own cars when they turn sixteen.

Fast forward to the past year of my life, when simple walking is an effort. It's Christmas Eve, and I am wondering where I will be a year from now, breaking the rule of staying in the present moment. *Don't even think about it.*

Fri, December 25, 2020
Covid Christmas Now Behind Us

We spent the day Zooming and doing Facetime with our children and grandchildren. Calls with siblings, etc. We are exhausted. We shared a great dinner, a bottle of Barolo, and called it quits around 10 pm. What the fuck! And there was none of that either.

*Dying is fine but Death, oh baby I wouldn't like
Death if Death were good*

—e.e. cummings

PART TWO

Chapter 14
NEW YEAR/NEW DEAL

January 2021: The Age of Acceptable Death
Musing as we enter a new year. If I die this year at the age of 77, once again, no one would say "Too young." Friends would smile and shake their heads, most likely remarking, "She had an incredible life!" And of course they would be right. We must embrace our mortality. Death is one of the few certainties of life.

Everybody dies—even though we were the generation that was going to live forever—so what would be considered an acceptable age or time? We don't get to pick that: life is a lottery, and we have lost too many friends in the last couple of years. But seeing my mother off at the age of 99 led me to the unreasonable belief that I would reach a ripe old age in pretty good health. As long as she was alive, I felt young and vibrant.

Despite the struggles of this past year, this morning I had the ultimate pleasure of a mile and a half walk around the bayfront, with the aid of my trekking pole and my lovely husband. How fortunate we both are.

Following Bill's accident he had been given a less than 20% chance of survival. He feels lucky every day just to be alive. "Every day is a gift!" is one of his often used expressions. He could be the *poster man* for living every day to the fullest. The past year, with my diagnosis and Covid affecting the world, I've had the time to truly reflect on what matters and let go of the rest. I am grateful for that. I still vow to clean out all my closets. I wouldn't want anyone else going through my stuff and knowing how messy I am. Pandemic isolation presented an unexpected gift—time to reflect and understand myself, my illness, and where I am going.

Creative Visualization and the Law of Attraction

Creative Visualization is using your imagination to picture goals and things you want to achieve in life. I'm hoping this still works when an unwelcome illness has entered the picture.

I remember all too well the self-help books of the seventies and eighties. I loved them and practiced what I read for about a month before moving on to the next trend. Now I'm thinking I should go back and try it again. I'll send my desire to be able to skip and climb stairs out into the universe. I'll visualize where I want to be in a year: attending the high school graduations of two grandsons, dancing at a nephew's wedding in Maine.

The first step is knowing my goal and believing it can

happen. And why shouldn't it? Bill says that as he lay in the ICU of Tampa Burn Center day after day, he always knew he would get better. He never doubted it.

So here I go. I Google and find a combo of the two techniques I'm looking for:

Uncover a powerful 4-step creative therapy exercise that will help you make rapid changes in your life. Use this exercise to improve a skill, change a habit, or improve your ability to manifest with the Law of Attraction. You choose the goal and then with practice, creative visualization will work its magic! Creative visualization helps you feel motivated and take inspired action, with less reliance on willpower.

This is the reason Creative Visualization works so effectively. When you vividly imagine the things you want in life, your brain and nervous system will believe that they already exist and will act accordingly.

(https://selfhelpforlife.com/)

Newly inspired. I'm not accepting the prognosis of continued muscle degeneration. My beliefs about me will change. It will change my sense of who I am and what I can do. For now, I can't skip or hop; but I begin visualizing myself wearing a low-heeled boot instead of sneakers. I wonder if this will work.

It's only four steps. Do this every day for a few months. Do it in the morning.

Mon, January 18, 2021 A Good Choice

Courage, according to the Merriam-Webster Dictionary, is a noun meaning the ability to do something that frightens one: "She called on all her courage to face the ordeal" or strength in the face of pain or grief: "He fought his illness with great courage."

According to Wikipedia, **courage** (also called **bravery** or **valor**) is the choice and willingness to confront agony, pain, danger, uncertainty, or intimidation. **Physical courage** is bravery in the face of physical pain, hardship, even death or threat of death.

Courage is the *choice* and *willingness* to confront agony, pain, danger, uncertainty, or intimidation.

It doesn't really feel like a choice, but I guess it's never too late to develop new habits.

Life's School of War

In 1888, German philosopher Friedrich Nietzsche first stated, "Out of life's school of war—what doesn't kill me, makes me stronger." This sentence has become an overused aphorism, but nevertheless accurately portrays a picture of resilience and offers an affirmation for overcoming adversity. I believe this. But I will still mourn the loss of being able to wear beautiful footwear.

Mon, February 1, 2021

Time moves slowly during the pandemic. I'm trying to "go with the flow" but feel frustrated much of the time. Bill suggests I talk to Rona about my mortality issues. "I did, but she said she'd rather focus on *living*." I sometimes slip into the "Why Me?" And I think of wearing myself out with my mother and flash to the questions "Why did I do it? Why wasn't I strong enough to stand up for myself in the situation?" She didn't appreciate anything I did, and my family took me for granted because I was the only sibling who lived in close proximity. Today, I have the answer from Rona. "You are a good human being! Move on."

Thurs, February 4, 2021 Psychotherapist

It's been a little over a year since I've been living with my Inclusion Body Myositis diagnosis. I do not know if I'm progressing…hard to tell on a day-to-day basis. I do know that my foot neuropathy, if anything, has gotten worse and walking is difficult. Because we are still in the pandemic and not going out much, I think about it a lot—too much— and then my mind floods with anxiety about my future. Bill looks forward to when we can travel again; I fear it. I am trying not to visualize myself in a wheelchair at the airport pre-boarding.

In the absence of having something to look forward to, I "recycle garbage—it's like looking in a rearview mirror instead of out the windshield." I love that! But now we are scheduled for the Covid vaccine, and then I will be able to get to Baltimore to Johns Hopkins and possibly the clinical drug trial. If I get the drug and not the placebo and it works, it will stop the muscle degeneration. Then I can rebuild muscle and stabilize. It will be good, and it is something to look forward to.

I am practicing becoming more **assertive** with people. This comes from a position of "I," and it's positive. Aggressive is when you are pointing the finger and is way less effective—at least that is what Rona has told me.

I let go of things that don't make me happy; then I have more room for things that do.

Sat, February 6, 2021

I write to Dr. Expert's assistant, a lovely and caring nurse, expressing my frustrations at being in a holding position. Not in control. She responds:

Dear Susan:

I can only sympathize with the frustration you are experiencing with IBM. I worked with Multiple Sclerosis patients for many years at Walter Reed Army Medical Center. I found that in many ways living with a debilitating disease is much like going through a grieving process. You must grieve the loss of who you were before you can accept the reality of who you have become. Neither is superior to the other; they are just different. Many of my MS patients use the phrase, "I have MS. MS doesn't have me" as their mantra. Somehow, that statement is empowering and can restore a sense of control over one's life. I would encourage you to proclaim that you have IBM. IBM does not have you! Know that you are not alone. I am here if and when you need to talk. If you believe that "It takes a village to raise a child," then you also know that "It takes a medical village to conquer a disease." We are here whenever you need us.

Namaste

And those heartfelt and profound words and wisdom from someone I've met once, mean more can I can possibly express. I feel blessed. I have IBM but it doesn't have me!

*The life you have led doesn't need
to be the only life you have.*

—Anna Quindlen

Sat, February 27, 2021   Hopeful

We are scheduled for our second vaccine in two days. I have resumed pestering Johns Hopkins regarding acceptance in their upcoming clinical drug trial. If I can't beat this IBM, can I be a beacon of hope for others? After all, it's not the moments that define us, but how we respond to them. A combination of curiosity and tenacity and a positive attitude.

The Problem

Bill says my problem is stress—that I go looking for it, it's free-floating, and I will always find it. "Talk to Rona about your always being stressed."

Thurs, March 4, 2021   Rona Today

My feelings get hurt, and I am very sensitive. It's a recreation of my dynamic with my mother. Why do I give people power to hurt my feelings?

Dredging up the past has always been a favorite pastime of mine: I punish myself with the retrospectoscope. My doctor friend says I have achieved Olympic class status. It is exhausting and brings nothing good along with it. It's old stuff. I pull out the resentment tapes and press play. Rona reminds me yet again that we cause our own suffering when we dwell on things that hurt us. I must change the story that I'm sensitive and thin-skinned.

But is it possible to alter the human condition? To transform? To unburden from and heal childhood trauma? *Grow the fuck up and move forward.* This I say to myself. Rona never uses swear words. But Rona short-times me. And

I have a fear of powerful women, which I have discussed with her, so I'm hesitant to mention it, even meekly. Today I say, "How much time do I have with you?" I always feel rushed at the end of a session. She tells me 50 minutes. I freeze, because she cuts me off at no later than 45 minutes and she bills for 60 minutes. So here I am with a woman I'm intimidated by as my therapist and I am afraid to say how I feel. She accepts Medicare, so I am grateful.

Plot Point

If this were a movie, today would have been a plot point: something unexpected happens that takes the story and turns it around in another direction. Every movie has two key plot points.

I am trying to set myself up at Hopkins and my hoped-for cure. I have called several people who are involved in coordinating the trial and finally am told by a young woman: Oh hi, the trial has been put off till the fall. "When in the fall, September, October, November? Why?" Blah blah blah.

It's out of my control. Then I see there is a professor at Tel Aviv University who has a drug primarily for Covid-19 that seems to have other good effects, like bringing down inflammation and helping autoimmune disease. I Google him and get his email, then write to him.

"So, we're going to Israel?" Bill says. "I love it."

I get a response from the professor a few hours later.

Dear Susan
You are a wise woman
In theory I tend to say yes
However we do not have any clue if our drug has
any systemic
absorption from the lung
I suggest you to contact MSD (oncoimmune) and
try their
CD24FC drug that is being given by the IV route

Thanks
Nadir

I am beyond impressed that he has written back. Aided by an adrenalin rush, I write back and ask where I can get the other drug. The company has been sold to Merck, and I see it is being tested at NIH, where Dr. Expert heads the myositis department. I send the information to him and wait for a response.

At a certain age and stage in life, you realize there isn't an infinite amount of time left to do something meaningful with your talents. The shorter that timeline grows, the greater the sense of urgency to do something that might leave the world a better place for your having been in it.

Hinterland: An area lying beyond what is visible or known, or Looking for Loopholes

Bill is an extraordinarily good joke teller and he seems to have an anecdote for just about every occasion. One such story is about the American comedian, actor, and writer W.C. Fields, a confirmed atheist. On his deathbed, he was visited by a couple of his old buddies, who found him reading a bible. One friend asked why, as a known nonbeliever, he was now reading the bible. Field's alleged answer: "Looking for loopholes!"

I am a fallen away Roman Catholic—a post-Catholic. I am spiritual but not fond of organized religion that was so forced down my throat along with the cruciferous vegetables in my growing years: I developed a disdain for both.

Today I had a doctor's appointment on the pretense of asking for a prescription for Physical Therapy but mostly to vent and have her view my rapid physical decline. Over the weekend I had read a book by my old friend, legendary author Dan Wakefield, called *Is It God?* Formerly I had been turned off by this wonderful writer and storyteller's switch from best-selling books-to-movies to spiritual books, although I had never read his recent books. Surprisingly, he wove his usual humorous prose into the points he was making, and it was as entertaining as all of his other books. I was sitting in the doctor's office, thinking, *God, and Raphael* (archangel of healing), *can you give me a sign?* I'm not sure what kind of sign or why, but I needed a sign.

An hour later, prescription for PT in hand, I was at Whole Foods feeling, okay, yes—sorry for myself, my exhaustion, my blurry vision and sense of imbalance. Someone, caftan-dressed and wearing a head turban, stood in front of me with their shopping cart and was taking what seemed an inordinately long time removing an item from the glassfront refrigerator. I waited patiently and then as I passed, I saw a terribly scarred burn victim with a rebuilt, stretched and shiny nose and mouth opening and no ears-the hands webbed.

I took this as a sign. There is always someone in worse shape, and this could have been my husband, who suffered third-degree burns on a third of his body. His face was spared, mercifully; he had great plastic surgeons at Tampa Burn Center; and he healed. How lucky we both are. Feeling gratitude.

My situation propels me to continue to look for loopholes. Today, massage therapist shows me a Hyperice vyper vibrating roller for $200. "Your body will like this, put your feet on it!" She also says the nerve repair vitamins work and she can sell them to me as well as the lavender oil: "Your body likes the calming effect." I buy it all. I am not insane, but this is where desperation takes us: the chronically ill, the weak, the hopeless. We are forced to find hope. Healing by any means. Healing against all odds. I can dream and I hope for miracles.

Rona listens to my story and states flatly that massage therapists should not be selling products.

Sun, March 21

We're having Sunday breakfast and reading the *NY Times*. It has a story about a horse retreat in New Mexico "that offers a hard-to-define experience that may include a joyful rewiring of one's brain." I'm reading it to Bill over coffee. "No," he says. "Stop this insanity."

We are fully vaccinated, and this makes us feel safe. I can see my daughter and grandchildren, whom I have not seen since a year ago last Christmas: one year and three months. They are coming to visit next week.

The New Simpatico/The New Me

"Living with a debilitating disease is much like going through a grieving process. You must grieve the loss of who you were before you can accept the reality of who you have become," said the nurse at Hopkins. So it's not acceptance, but more a reality check that my life has changed, at least for the moment, and I must adapt. I am a devotee of fashion footwear including mid heels for special occasions, but my body says, "No more." My illness has messed with my identity and having to wear flats is just more bad news. Is there such a thing as chic flats or sneakers? I know it sounds shallow, but the strapped Mary Jane style alternate does not complement my social wardrobe and flats don't give the height equity and ensuing confidence of a smart looking pair of pumps. I suddenly have to change my look because of my disease and that is completely out of my control. But safety rules and I must keep my two feet planted firmly on the ground.

I will probably never be what I was—and that propels me to give away my good shoes with low to high heels that I love but can no longer wear. It's like saying goodbye to old and dear friends. A tearful departure. Despite my neuropathy vitamins, exercise, and vibrating foot roller, I am unable to even stand in any of my prized pumps, sandals and boots. Walking would be an impossibility. I offer some of the highest and sexiest models to my slim and stylish fiftyish Pilates instructor. She is thrilled and tells me they fit her as though they were custom made for her feet by the master of footwear, Salvatore Ferragamo. This is truly joyful news!

My biggest fear is going from a life of independence to one of dependency; this is what I am fighting against and is also why I am always exhausted. The B12 injections offer no significantly impact my energy level—another lost friend—even if it was nervous energy.

So I am struggling—yet vertical. I have much to be grateful for.

I think back to so many years ago, when Bill and I, in our late forties, had been married just five years. His lovely mother, athletic and an avid golfer, lived nearby. It was a shock when she was given a terminal cancer diagnosis at the age of 72. I remember thinking that was old. But she was a widow, and despite having four loving children, I'm sure she felt alone and helpless during her remaining months. We moved her in with us and made her comfortable, and Bill made her laugh. But she was not ready to die. I'm five years older than she was. Neither am I.

Chapter 15
OSKIE!

Fri, April 23, 2021

I finally addressed the adnexal cysts that showed up on the MRI on my trip to NIH in January of 2020. Today, fifteen months later, was the ultrasound, and I am waiting for the results. It's Friday, and I have called the office because the doctor was in but the nurse said he may not get a chance to look at the results until Monday. So will I spend the weekend worrying about whether I have ovarian cancer while GYN is on his boat? No! So I make a second plea to the office to please call me back with the results before the end of the day.

The call at 4:34 pm Friday: Cysts on ovaries are small, simple cysts. No intervention necessary. You can follow up in six months. Again, I feel like Woody Allen's character in the movie *Annie Hall* (back when I liked Woody), when he finds out he doesn't have brain cancer and he leaves the doctor's office, jumping and clicking his heels together.

I can't do that now, but still can't help the feeling that I dodged another bullet.

Reflections

Oh how happy I am that we have traveled far and wide; we didn't wait. At times I was resentful because I had book tours going on and grandbabies about to be born and thought I should be elsewhere—and we were constantly on the go. Now I feel so grateful and fortunate to have done this.

Along the way we listened to so many people who said, "We're going to do what you're doing, when we retire." Guess how many people didn't make it? Too many weren't able to realize their dream. We had the joie de vivre and sense of adventure and associated acceptance of risk to pursue our goals.

Inevitable Changes

We have shifted from movers and shakers to early birds. We sit outside once a week at our favorite restaurant, Mediterraneo in Sarasota. Our former 8pm reservation has changed to 6—or even 5:30. You'd think we had retired to Florida.

Setback Sunday—May 2, 2021

We set off on our first trip since Covid prevented us from going anywhere. We're only going one hour away to visit my youngest brother (by fifteen years) and his wife in Englewood, Florida. We are silly and excited. "Road Trip!" Bill says with great enthusiasm as we load up the car. A sense of freedom takes over as we—the fully vaccinated—feel the cloud of doom has been lifted.

So happy to see and hug family. We sit and chat and catch up.

They are boaters and own two large boats, so the first order of the day is a sunset cruise. They have packed a cooler with snacks and drinks, and brother assures me I will have no problem getting onto their pontoon boat. There is a steep step to the dock, and Bill and my brother somehow lift me down. We walk to the boat to find the tide has risen, lifting the boat up a foot. This makes it impossible for me to board, as the boat is now a foot above the dock as well as a jump across. We stand and look at each other. Bill says, "Sorry guys, she can't do it. We can't risk anything happening before we get to Hopkins in three weeks." Everyone is kind and understanding, so we go and sit on their lanai—me feeling like I ruined the day.

But I didn't. We had fun watching the Kentucky Derby and making bets, and they served a delicious chicken parmesan dinner. We stayed up late talking, till I finally went to bed at 11:30. The toilet in the bathroom was low, and they offered me the use of the new, higher model in their bathroom. I thanked them and said I'd be fine.

Sunday morning around 10:30, I go for a quick pee before leaving. I had managed (barely) the toilet since we'd been there, but I was tired. "If you need me, here's the code," Bill says- "Oskie, Oskie!" "Huh?" "It means interception."*

I try to push myself up from the toilet, holding onto the sink, and I am unable to get up. I try again and again and again, but the quadricep muscles will not fire. I reach for the towel bar on the wall in front of me and wonder if I will pull it off the ceramic tile if I can reach it. I start to shake, and my quads are shaking. "Bill," I call out, not remembering his code or even knowing where he might be in the house, or even outside, wondering if he could even hear me. Louder, "Bill! *Bill!*"

Mercifully he arrives. He faces me, puts his arms under my arms as we have practiced, and pulls me up from sitting to standing. My entire body is still shaking. This is a major setback. Major fears are stairs and toilets. We have a problem! I need his help physically and emotionally. I never signed up to not be able to get up from the toilet. Neither did he. UGH!

***Oskie**
When an interception takes place in football, the player who intercepted the ball shouts **"oskie"** to alert his teammates. The team then reverses direction and blocks for the player who intercepted the ball, clearing the way for the interception return.

May 2021   Toilet Hack from Nurse

Dear Susan,
How exciting that you are being considered for a clinical drug trial. I do not know the doctor personally, but do know him by reputation, which is stellar.
I can understand your apprehension with travel. I have taken two separate trips to South Carolina

and Florida to help bring my daughter home. Both trips were pre-vaccines. The airports were ghost towns. People were cordial and respectful, but the airport and the airplanes all had an eerie energy about them. I tested each time I returned and thankfully came up negative. All in my household have been double vaccinated.

I can understand your concerns about toilets. (My mother used to say that I had dragged her into every single restroom in the world. Some only had a hole in the ground and two footprints.) In order to help you get up off the public restroom toilets, you may consider carrying a length of strong nylon cord, long enough to loop around the top of a stall door and reach you on the toilet. (Nylon cord is lightweight and can be hidden easily in your purse.) The loop around the door should be a slip knot, making it adjustable. You could also loop the slip knot around a purse hook on the door. The end that you hold while on the toilet would have a fixed loop/handle. When you are ready to stand up, you pull the cord, using it as leverage to help you up. NB: Make sure you have securely locked the door!! And your feet are planted firmly on the floor. Practice at using a chair positioned in front of a door. See if it works for you! Let me know if you try it.

Sat, May 8, 2021

Another tired day. Went out last night with good friends. Forgot my distance glasses as well as the usual half an Ativan for social activities and Pepcid for reflux. Went to bed at 11. Think my body is giving up on me. I am no longer any semblance of the former me. Yet somehow I persist as I walk into Dillard's with the aid of a cane. I'm grateful I can walk.

Later today we have Dr. Z for his long-awaited visit at the studio at 4 pm, followed by an unplanned-for (Bill says we have to go to) dinner—friends of friends visiting from Boston. Still trying to figure out how to navigate my fatigue and difficulty walking. Formerly enjoyable social dinners have become the ultimate challenge.

According to my "Angel Visionary" reading:

"It can be easy to fall into a pattern of negative words, thoughts, and emotions but your angels are here to remind you that you attract what you broadcast into the Universe and to what degree. Fretting and sweating about nightmare scenarios will attract that outcome to you, so be careful with what you say and think."

Okay, thanks. I guess I needed a reminder. There will be a drug and I will get better. I've got this!

Thurs, May 13, 2021
Final Visit with Rona before we leave for Baltimore and then Boston

I want to talk about being a burden to Bill, but in doing so, I realize I am mad at him for insisting we have friends to dinner tonight. I try to explain it takes too much energy to entertain at home, and he says it's not really a dinner--he will cook burgers. We don't have a grill and I still have to do all the work. "We'll sit outside," he says. "You don't have to do a Martha Stewart." "Penis brain!" I say to Rona. She tells me to make an agreement—to revisit it and stick to it.

I tell her I am dizzy and off balance, and the mere act of walking is difficult for me. She gives me a tangible tip in an effort to try to get Bill to understand my balance issues and what it feels like. "Buy a box of corkscrew rigatoni pasta and put some in his shoes and tell him to walk. This is what walking feels like to you, all the time, every day. He'll probably get it."

Also: "Focus on you and make healthy choices your priority. One day at a time, one event at a time. Don't project into the future. Be mindful."

We return to the subject of my mother, who has now been gone from this planet for three years. She is still in my head as the cause of my current situation. Rona tells me to "change the channel" when this happens, but this I have not yet mastered. I'll try harder.

I take half of a Pepcid and get ready for our guests. Have I mentioned that now when I drink sparkling water or red wine I get a forceful case of the hiccups? Bill tells me the rain has stopped so we can sit outside and it's going to be a great night.

Of course, he's right. Our friends arrive, and we are happy to see them. When the boys are inside getting drinks, my friend asks how I am doing and also if the doctors know how I got this Inclusion Body Myositis. I tell her that the acupuncturist attributed it to heavy stress. According to Johns Hopkins research:

It's possible that autoimmune disease occurs based on the immune system's ability to handle stress. Dr. Orbai says that this is an area of intense research. "When does the stress on your body exceed your immune system's ability to handle it? If we knew this, it could be the key to preventing autoimmune disease before it develops."

I tell her a few stories about the last five years of my mother's life, which include: my many attempts to get her to stop driving, the numerous visits to the hospital and rehab, her demands and her nastiness—her continuous expectations of me, the only daughter. Often I could actually feel chemical changes at the end of some stressful days spent with Mom and I knew it was toxic. My friend listened intently: "You have to get rid of all that, because it's still there! You have to vomit it all out in order to go forward with your life and get better." Hmm. Maybe she is on to something. We need a new rite for exorcism of a deceased family member-her ghost. The practice of expelling demons from a person has not been of obvious concern to the Catholic Church.

May 15, 2021

On further consideration I do not think my body could withstand an exorcism. I think I will try clemency. Maybe Rona was right when she said, "She's dead, go forward." I forgive you, Mom; I tried my best, even though it never seemed enough.

When I think about my mother's life story it makes me understand that we all arrive at a place from somewhere. As the youngest of six children, she was treated by her parents and siblings with a general disrespect or disregard; For example, she wasn't allowed to go to college because her mother was saving the money for her brothers. She was so religious that she never questioned her mother or the teachings of the Church. As I understand more of where she came from, I find a deeper level of compassion.

Forgiveness is letting go of pain, accepting what happened and releasing it. Forgiveness is not for the other person, it's for you. When you forgive you become free: when you let go you start to grow.

Oddly, I'd probably do the same thing all over again with a few exceptions. I would manage the stress better and taken the Ativan prescription I got from my doctor. Then I wouldn't have to be taking it now. And I wouldn't have felt the need to re-live every event with nightly updates to all my relatives thereby re- recreating the stress.

I owe much to my mother. After all, she gave birth to me—which I was repeatedly told was a long and difficult one. She prayed the rosary for a full day and to the Blessed Mother—hence my middle name, Marie. I finally arrived.

More recently, she gave me a second life. Bill and I travel together 99% of the time. We hire a car service to and from the airport. In the back seat, he sits behind the driver on the left and I sit on the right. If I had been in the car with him as planned on the way from Tampa Airport to Sarasota in August of 2016, when the driver lost his brakes and the car filled with black smoke and then fire, neither of us would have made it. But I had come home three days earlier to complete the sale of my mother's house and have the staging furniture removed, which is why I was not in the car.

I imagine if I had been with him, my first thought would have been to tell the story with great drama, including all details—first black smoke, then loss of brakes, finally fire. Almost unconsciously I became a storyteller. My last thought or ability might have been to dive headfirst out of the speeding, burning car onto the highway. But Bill wouldn't have fled the car without me, so neither of us would have survived—sadly, the driver did not. As it really happened, with superhuman capacity and bravery, Bill's first instinct was to dive out. He is Superman, and we are beyond grateful for the bonus years we have shared.

Thurs, May 20, 2021   Getting Ready for Baltimore

Here we go; the long awaited trip for evaluation is finally here. I am unable to do all the walking so we have the first wheelchair experience at the airport, and I'm convinced everyone is staring at me.

We will be here for five days, and our second day requires getting a Covid test and spending more than six hours in the hospital before meeting with Dr. Expert. I have to get him to like me so I can be accepted into the upcoming clinical trial. We spend the weekend because biopsies are only done on Monday. The doctor has ordered just one biopsy from my left bicep and nothing from my thigh. This is good news.

Mon, May 24, 2021

5 am wake-up call for Uber ride to outpatient surgery at Hopkins.

Sit and wait till someone retrieves us around 6:15 to fill out yet more of the same paperwork and answer the same Covid questions that these office people must be so tired of asking and I am extremely tired of answering. Have you been out of the country in the past six months? Have you been in contact with anyone who has Covid?

Nurse leads me to pre-surgery after giving Bill my pocketbook, wallet, wedding ring, watch, and earrings. I may never see him again.

Nurse hands me two gowns. "Everything off including underwear. One gown goes on opening in back, one opening in front." Doc arrives. Young and funny. I like him. Everyone is so careful, and surgeon explains procedure. "Incision this big." He demonstrates with his thumb and forefinger of his right hand. "You agreed to research, right?" He will take two biopsies for him, and if there is enough he will take a third for the research mouse.

Next I walk to where doc and assistant are waiting for first surgery of the day. It's 7:30, right on schedule. I am lying on the operating table on my back as they strap my left arm to a gurney board. I make a fist a few times so he can see the muscle where he will cut. He explains. They build a sterile tent between my arm and my face so I don't see the surgery. They begin by asking me what music I would like. Dylan or Bocelli would suit me. No rap, please. I've heard more rap music in the Uber cars in the city of Baltimore in the past few days than in my entire life.

The surgical area is cleansed and then numbed with local anesthetic. He cuts and explains. I'm thinking I feel very confident with these two MDs. One guy asks what I do, and I tell him I used to write relationship books and do television and radio talk shows and I was on Oprah. Three nurses come to an abrupt halt and gape at me in awe, or so it seems behind the masks. "You were on Oprah? Omg." Always the same reaction when I tell people I appeared on *Oprah* as a relationship expert. "What is she like?" The procedure takes a little over an hour, and I go to recovery. "No pressure on left arm for 48 hours. Stitches are dissolvable. No shower for three days."

Bill arrives from the outside courtyard to recovery, where I am now dressed and waiting, left arm in sling.

Macho guy walking around with my Fendi striped tote bag with red handle over his shoulder. So sweet. I'm wondering how I will get up from a chair or the toilet with the use of only one arm. My quads alone won't do it, I know for sure.

After a stop at Starbucks we return to hotel sip our cappuccino. Now the intense aching pain kicks in. Bill goes to drugstore to buy the recommended Tylenol. But we're done.

Later

So now we know there is no cure and no current drug trial. How do I feel? How am I? Do I start the grieving again? Or the fighting process? Or do I remain in a state of pissed-off-ness?

I've had a good run. As Bill has begun to remind me, I will be 78 on my next birthday. Wow, the number is shocking. My mother was in good shape and still driving at age 94. I am not my mother. But—and I don't mean this in a complaining way—this occurred around the time of her death, when Bill had miraculously recovered from his accident and we were so grateful, and then due to the diligence of my attorney brother, who was the executor, I actually received my birthright in a timely manner after my mother passed away. I was on a roll, or so I thought.

Life is what happens when you're busy making other plans.

— John Lennon

Chapter 16
THE VERDICT IS IN

Fri, May 28, 2021
A Scintilla of Hope—Why Not?

Dr. Expert says he is 99% sure of the diagnosis; "The muscle biopsy is the gold standard, but we get few surprises." Daughter doctor has insisted on this biopsy from the onset. Daughter is smart, solid, steady, and straightforward—never invasive. So I have always hung my hope on the muscle biopsy showing a lesser disease with an available cure. *I want more!* I tell the universe.

The surgeon said he was only 56% convinced that I had IBM because some things did not match up: muscle enzymes were not that high. "I want a miracle," I tell him. "Well," he continued, "IBM is not the worst disease."

My mother in her final year would say, "I ask the Lord to take me every day," yet she fought, did not miss a meal, got her hair done weekly, and did her crossword puzzles religiously. I ask the Lord to give me another shot at life and I promise to enjoy every second I can walk and get out of a chair or up from a toilet. Please, God! I'll be an advocate for handicapped toilets everywhere.

And so we wait for the results, which may come today, Friday, but it is Memorial Day weekend, and after analysis of results, which is supposed to be today, the docs must write up their notes and post them on my chart, so it may be another week before I know my fate. I'll enjoy my days of hopefulness. Breathe deeply and exhale with my navel touching my backbone! Enjoy being in Boston, despite the fact that it is cold and rainy, and enjoy seeing our children, grandkids, and relatives. Inhale calm! I am so fortunate!

Sat, May 29, 2021   The New Reality Hits

It's Saturday afternoon as we head south out of Boston to visit daughter and family in Hingham. They have a beautiful and comfortable home, which we have not been to since Christmas 2019, when I was in better shape. The Uber driver drops us off, and I scan the different entrances—all with stairs. Bill suggests we walk over the grass to flat entrance with one small step. All good.

Anxiety hits as I wonder whether, if I need to use the bathroom, I will be able to get up from the toilet. We check it out, and I think I can manage.

When leaving four hours later, after a lovely and relaxing dinner, we call Uber and decide to try the stairs; it's easier to go down than up, and it's dark out. Bill holds tightly to my still sore biopsied left arm. We had brought laundry with us and packed it in a carry-on with rollers.

The bottom step is steep, so Bill puts the roller bag on the driveway and turns to lift me down the bottom stair, just as the roller bag takes off rolling down the driveway towards the street. Fortunately he is able to rescue it just before the Uber driver pulls in. Narrow escape all around.

My new reality becomes painfully apparent as I try to maneuver the most ordinary situations: getting out of different model cars, small slants on floors, steep steps—general walking and feeling any semblance of balance. Today I took one teaspoon (5 grams) of creatine powder, as suggested by Dr. Expert at Hopkins. I did not read the directions and added it to my morning coffee, and was hyper all day. I finally read the directions which said: Mix with water or juice. Do not use with caffeine. I am discouraged.

Sun, May 30, 2021   Looking for Signs

Whenever I read about guardian angels, it says that they surround you and will help you, and to be open to signs—a feather, a rainbow, a certain color. As a former Catholic, that is the only religion I am familiar and comfortable with, even in my discomfort with organized religion in general. I'm looking for signs when I turn on my computer to check emails and I see that I have 1,111 unread emails. My adored father died at the age of 84 on 11/11 in the year 2000. This must be a sign: I've been praying to him for help. I know he has heard me. He is my connection to God.

I remember back to my fall off the commuter train in Siena three and a half years ago, and my first cosmetically driven thought was that they would have to shave my newly highlighted hair in order to stitch the deep gash where I hit the back of my head on the concrete platform. Lucky for me they did not.

A few weeks later, squatting down to get something, I dropped to the ground on the cobblestone street of Florence and found that I was completely unable to get up. Little did I know it was the beginning of something chronic. All the annoying clichés I grew up hearing were beginning to make perfect sense: *As long as you have your health*; *you can't take it with you.*

It's cold and rainy in our beautiful rental apartment on the Boston waterfront. The heat was turned off and switched to just AC on May 15. It's raw—like Florence in November. We decide to snuggle in and watch *City on the Hill,* a Showtime drama set in Boston. Partway through my iPhone dings.

4:10 Sunday: The Verdict

I am shocked to receive a new and unexpected email message from Johns Hopkins. There is a new lab result waiting on the My Chart page.

We are watching the show. Bill asks if I want to check it. "No."

I was expecting nothing till Tuesday earliest. I start to shake, then deep-breathe. Panic. Anxiety, my fate. I'll probably have a stroke waiting for the biopsy results.

6:00 pm; the show is over. I walk to the computer—Bill beside me-- and open My Chart from email with trembling fingers. What could it say? I have IBM; or I have something worse? What stage is it? No more hope!

I click test results. Covid test required for surgery: negative. I knew that and click lab results, but there is nothing.

*You only live once, but if you do it right,
once is enough.*

— Mae West

Chapter 17
WAITING

Tues, June 1, 2021   Supplements and Other Stuff

Day 8 post-surgery. Still in Boston. Still no word on the biopsy. Dr. Expert did recommend creatine powder daily to help build muscle. I ordered it from Amazon, and today is day 5 of using it properly. I'm reading a lot about nutrition and chronic diseases.

Bill is out visiting grandchildren, and I am not confident going out on my own. Google beckons me, and I can't resist. I watch a video on MS and how this woman Pam says she was cured and she is the living example. An email pops up from Dr. Gundry, who seems to have the same gut-related diagnosis for everything with an accompanying supplement. In listening, I realize he is not that far from the MS-recovered patient who claims that all these illnesses and infections come from the gut. His newest product is a powder dietary supplement, Primal Plants, a concentrated green polyphenol blend that supports skin health and optimizes energy and digestion. One scoop a day in an 8 oz. glass of water. I order it. Bill would say the last salesman would always win me, I am so gullible.

So now I take collagen powder in my morning coffee and creatine in water before I exercise, and somewhere I'll find a time for the new supplement that will help me poop and give me gorgeous skin and a healthier gut. Life is great!

Bill wants to extend our agreed-to time in Boston. Of course he does; he has most of his family members here, friends, all of his children and grandchildren, and many relatives. Because of my chronic fatigue and fear of toilet height, I am unable to do what I want. This left me alone yesterday, while he visited his daughter and three grand-kids, and I'll stay in again tonight, while he is having dinner with a great friend whose wife also is not up to dinner. She has stage 4 cancer.

So what do we do? Bill is having a ball. He wants to pay an extra $1,000 to change our tickets and stay at the beautiful apartment three more nights. We still have ten days to go as it is, and I'm ready to go home and get back to my routine. At least at home in Sarasota, I can drive to acupuncture, massage, and Pilates. It's not working for me. Doing a nosedive as I impatiently await the biopsy results.

Wed, June 2, 2021   High Anxiety

9 days post-op, and still no news. Wondering why I am so anxious. First of all, I'm afraid to get the report because it could definitively confirm my diagnosis of IBM, leaving

no possibility of a misdiagnosis. And secondly, it could be something worse—but possibly treatable? Based on my current condition and difficulty walking, climbing stairs, extreme fatigue—it's not nothing!

I don't know when I learned to pick up things with my toes, but I suspect it was as a preteen, when my five brothers and I would compete in all sorts of simple games—this being one I excelled at. Now, as I drop things on the floor and am unable to squat and lean to pick them up, I have adapted. Bill thinks it is beyond weird, comparing me to a monkey. Despite the fact that PT at Hopkins gifted me a stick to use, I prefer my toes and consider it a beneficial exercise.

Fri, June 4, 2021

11 days post-op. Running out of patience, I text the surgeon as well as Dr. Expert, inquiring about biopsy results. It's been almost two weeks, and my mind continues to play games and torture me with what-if's. They must know something at this point. I don't want to go through another weekend not knowing anything about my future.

Deep breaths, hold, and let out slowly to a count of what-the-fuck!

Unrelenting anxiety. Will it be the original diagnosis of 18 months ago of 99% certain IBM, or will it be worse? It couldn't be "in my head" because I've had two brain scans that turned up no problems. Still hoping for misdiagnosis and something curable, or at least treatable.

Thinking about three years ago, July 2018, when approaching my 75th birthday, we went to South Africa on safari, to wine country, and to Cape Town. We stayed at the Cape Grace in Cape Town, a hotel my father often spoke of as among his favorites. This trip I would not be able to manage now. We did a great deal of walking. I had difficulty climbing into the jeep, but managed with a shove up from Bill—but that was about it. My energy level was boundless, and it truly was the much dreamed of trip-of-a-lifetime: up close and personal with the elephants. Very grateful.

Life lesson that bears repeating: Never put off till retirement what you can do today—or you may never get to it.

Saturday morning, June 5, 2021

We are lying in bed, me sipping coffee at 8:30 in the morning. Bill strongly suggests that I text Dr. Expert again and explain why I am so anxious about getting the results of the "gold standard of diagnosis."

Within the hour, the long -awaited response arrives in my messages, along with a photo scan of biopsy slide and analysis.

Your muscle biopsy showed inflammatory cells invading muscle fibers and rimmed vacuoles. These are the hallmark features of IBM we wanted to prove you had. Any other questions?

Yeah, about a hundred, but mostly I'm disappointed. I was hoping and praying for a better outcome. So here I am, after 18 months of wondering—and now I know for sure. The slide report states that I have severe atrophy and biceps very weak. I had not known or anticipated this, and up until now have been focusing on strengthening my quadriceps. I need time to absorb this and form a plan.

When you have exhausted all possibilities,
remember this: you haven't.

—Thomas Edison

Going Forward:
Giving Up is Not an Option

My Pavlovian reaction is to go shopping. It's my cardio, my meditation, my relaxation. I love shopping; I can visualize endorphins releasing, the dopamine. But I can't manage the Boston stores unaccompanied; I am walking unsteadily, even with the aid of my cane.

Oh, how shopping was always my instant go-to stress relief—retail therapy. As the Joker said when going to rob, "When the going gets tough, the tough go shopping." I love the thrill of the purchase. The euphoria of the moment. I go for the next best thing and order groceries online to be delivered to our temporary quarters on the waterfront.

Whom do I tell of my definitively confirmed situation? My daughter-the-doctor first, and her husband. She responds that she is sorry to hear the results but it's good I finally know. I text a few close friends and relatives who have been caring and asking and waiting along with me. The responses immediately flood in, and I am too exhausted to continue texting. I don't want to talk to anyone and repeat the details. Bill suggests that I wait till Monday, saying "Nobody expects an answer over the weekend."

And so it goes. This is life; everyone gets something, and we're all on the same path, some going now at a speedier pace to the final destination and many with challenges along the way. Humans are planned obsolescence: we are all going to die. That's the set up! It's been preplanned by our creator. Out with the old—in with the new! It's important to make the most of what we have now.

Is it okay to text Rona? I won't be seeing her for a few weeks. What happened to my prayers and guardian angel intervention? Maybe it's coming in the form of a future drug trial acceptance.

This is a lifestyle change for Bill and me. No more late nights and maybe—if any—limited travel. The trip to Baltimore and Boston has been exhausting. I go to my favorite team at Sassoon on Boylston Street for my haircut and highlights. I have not seen them in a year and a half, and I decide to give them a Covid bonus tip of $100 each. I come back to the condo and check myself out in the mirror: hmm, the lined neck and thin face. I reach for the "Miracle Balm"—billed as "the secret of no-makeup makeup: a wash of soft-focus moisture to perfect and enhance skin," a recent purchase from Bobbi Brown's new moisturizing clean line of makeup called Jones Road. Dusty Rose cheeks: now at least I look healthier, and Bill always loves the look of my blown dry straight blonde hair.

In my young modeling days in my twenties, I worked with an older model, in her fifties, who had this expression: "A little powder and paint, makes a lady what she ain't." I'm remembering when I had to buy the "right outfit" before trying a new sport—I had to look the part. "It doesn't matter if you win or lose, but what you wear when you play the game." Shallow? Yep! Is it too late to change? Probably!

Sun, June 6, 2021   Big Yellow Taxi

Don't it always seem to go

That you don't know what you've got 'til it's gone?

They paved paradise
Put up a parking lot
Shoo, bop, bop, bop, bop
Shoo, bop, bop, bop, bop

Joni Mitchell was referring to the environment in her 1970s song—but the overall message is not taking things for granted. I took walking, climbing stairs, and getting up from a toilet as givens. I didn't know what I had till it was gone! The simple act of urination was never a *happening*.

Surrender is the simple but profound wisdom of yielding to rather than opposing the flow of life.

— Eckhart Tolle

Mon, June 7, 2021   Over and Next!

When Norman Lear, the prolific television producer, answered a recent Proust Questionnaire in *Vanity Fair* magazine, he was asked, "What is your motto?" He answered, **"Over and next.** When something is over, it is over, and we are on to next, and if there was a hammock in the middle of those two words that would be the best definition I know of living in the moment." "What is your idea of perfect happiness?" His response: "Waking up in the morning is as perfect as anything gets."

The Grieving Process.

Life has taken an unexpected turn. I am grieving a loss of something I thought I had for my lifetime—mobility. As I now hope for a cure, I will attempt to slow the muscle degenerative progress. I will pursue new information. Never underestimate the value of your own voice. I will be a participant in my own destiny.

I will also yield to the flow of life, exercise religiously, and see where it takes me. Oh yeah, and try not to worry about where we will be at Christmas. After all, it's only June. I feel better already! This is my new reality, and I will find the joy if it kills me.

Still in Boston, I realize we are one block away from James Hooks Waterfront Shanty on Atlantic Avenue, offering live lobsters in all forms. I am excited at the prospect of walking over with Bill and picking up the most delicious lobster roll in New England. It's all good!

*Trust in Science, Keep the Faith,
and Laugh More!*

—Alan Alda, American actor

PART THREE

Chapter 18
LIVING LIFE TO THE FULLEST

From What If to What Is

With a definitive diagnosis comes a new chapter. How it happened is less important than what happens now. The focus is on stability and stopping the progression. No sense in looking back; this is where we are! And it is very much "we;" Bill is a big part of this journey. The reality of the diagnosis has changed my approach from wondering to an all-out plan to enjoy every day, build strength, and stay vertical.

One thing that doesn't change is hope. Hope springs eternal. Maybe I'll have a new vocation in advocacy for IBM.

That said, what is realistic? Future travel? International travel? I was hoping my guardian angels would help me and I'd be able to dance my way out of this, but I still can't get my feet off the floor.

And There is Celebrity News

No effective treatment has been found so far for inclusion body myositis (IBM), a neurologic disorder that rock star Peter Frampton was diagnosed with in 2015, and several drugs have proved disappointing in clinical trials. "I'm very pragmatic about this disease and am always positive. I have to be," says Frampton. "IBM isn't *life-ending, it's life-altering*." It's always beneficial to have a celebrity attached to a chronic illness, as it will bring awareness and hopefully more funding for research, especially if it's not a popular or well-known disease. Peter Frampton says he found new purpose after his Inclusion Body Myositis diagnosis and was inspired to start a research foundation.

I see hope as the very heart of healing. For those who have hope, it may help some to love longer, and it will help all to live better. . . . Hope, I have come to believe, is as vital to our lives as the very oxygen we breathe.

—Jerome Groopman, M.D., *The Anatomy of Hope: How People Face Illness*

So What is Inclusion Body Myositis (IBM)?

"Myositis" refers to inflammation of muscle, and "inclusion body" refers to abnormal protein clumps within empty spaces called vacuoles that are visible in biopsied muscle cells. According to Dr. Lisa Christopher-Stine, head of the myositis clinic at Johns Hopkins: Muscles usually affected by IBM include the quadriceps, which help lock the knee and provide power while walking up steps. Lack of strength in these muscles can trigger falls, which is often why people go see a doctor. IBM also affects finger flexors, the forearm muscles that enable finger movement and dexterity. "Movements that involve grabbing objects—like turning a car key, using a screwdriver, holding utensils, or turning a doorknob—often become more difficult. . . . Ultimately, it becomes debilitating."

IBM has no available treatment or cure. The cause is unclear and continues to be debated. Inflammation suggests IBM is an autoimmune disorder, in which the immune system attacks healthy tissue. Yet drugs usually prescribed for autoimmune disorders, such as corticosteroids and immunosuppressants, tend to have little or no effect against IBM.

Does Everything Happen for a Reason?

Aristotle believed that everything happening to you today has a purpose because it turns you into the person you are becoming. Acceptance of this theory meshes with Eckhart Tolle's philosophy of surrender—yielding rather than opposing the flow of life. Go-with-the-flow and flourish becomes an empowering principle in my life. It's up to me to create meaning from all this as I accept my fate. Acceptance! I have now reached the final stage of grief!

As the Austrian neurologist, psychoanalyst, and Holocaust survivor Viktor Frankl says in his book *Man's Search for Meaning,* "Everything can be taken from a man but one thing: the last of the human freedoms—to choose one's attitude in any given set of circumstances, to choose one's own way."

There must be humor in this.

I was born the second child and only daughter of six children. My older brother died of lung cancer at the age of 70. Bill often reminds me: "You've got seven years on him." It was beyond painful to watch him suffer, yet he remained brave and dignified in his final emaciating months. I remember him telling me he had no bucket list and that he and his wife had recently taken up golf. And of course, I am next in lineal order. But in the end, he too was looking for loopholes. As a fallen-away Catholic, he thought it may be a good idea to get the last rites of the Catholic Church, just in case. This entails receiving the final sacrament of the Eucharist, which acts as viaticum (Latin, "provision for a journey"). Communion in the body and blood of Christ, received at this moment of "passing over" to the Father, has a particular significance and importance to a Catholic.

The fact that I recently took up golf does not escape me. Now I am unable to squat and bend far enough to tee up the ball, and Bill insists on helping out. This is when the term "What's your handicap?" takes on a new meaning. Onward!

"God Will Never Give you More Than You Can Handle."

This was the mantra of my devout Roman Catholic mother during tough times. If that failed, she'd say "Offer it [the pain] up to the suffering souls in purgatory." This usually occurred at the dentist, as we children were never allowed Novocain because of her fear of needles. If you did not grow up with the Baltimore Catechism—a storied old teaching tool of Christian Doctrine—and my mother as your spiritual guide, you probably won't get this. Okay, then, bring it on! I'll figure out how to handle it. Out with the WHY and in with the HOW! It's all about attitude and dealing with what is. Frankl also said, "When we are no longer able to change a situation, we are challenged to change ourselves."

*Just when the caterpillar thought
the world was over, it became a butterfly.*

—Chuang Tzu

Chapter 19
THE NEW NORMAL

The past has only the past to offer. The present is a time where new things can be experienced, improved, invented.

According to Wikipedia, *the New Normal* may refer to "the prevailing situation following widespread crisis." After the hopes and worries, Bill and I are navigating our way to a whole new normal. That's how Doctor Daughter refers to our situation: "Your new normal."

The Newly Changing Me

There are people I love and connect with, and I don't want to leave them yet—my husband and our children and grandchildren are at the top of this list. I am grateful for them and the wonderful years Bill and I have had together as we approach our 32nd anniversary next week. I have much to live for *but* I also want to outlive a few people—who shall remain nameless on these pages. I muster up the courage to change my perspective.

The Plan: Be happy and live a good life

I need to learn how to focus and to prioritize what matters most to me and let go of the rest. This is definitely going to take practice! Oh, the time wasted on insignificant events and people that don't matter. What matters? Family, friends, my health, purpose.

It's now me first and focused! How liberating!

Back to the Italian proverb and my new mantra: *Chi va piano, va sano e va lontano.* Those who go slowly, go in good health and go far. It's never too late to implement this school of thought—even with a chronic disease. It's time for your empowered self-healing to rise.

Many autoimmune patients are stuck in an identity of sickness. While they dream of being healthy again, the obstacle of going from sickness to health keeps them spinning their wheels. Like me, they have tried just about every conventional and/or holistic treatment out there, including various drugs and vitamins.

I admit to being overwhelmed and frustrated, and last year's whittled-down list of supplements has begun to expand again. It occurs to me that some may even contradict each other. Time to get back to basics!

Thurs, June 10, 2021

Just when I felt like I had successfully stopped chasing the next cure, I awake this morning to an email from a good and concerned friend. She attaches a link to a 2020 research study done on an IBM patient in New Zealand: *Impact of a Ketogenic Diet on Sporadic Inclusion Body Myositis: A*

Case Study. I read the study with new hope and interest and immediately forward it to Dr. Expert at Hopkins. What if this could slow down the progression?

Ketogenic diets are theoretically capable of suppressing inflammation, enhancing cell bioenergetics, alleviating mitochondria dysfunction, and stimulating autophagy, which may be beneficial in IBM. We report the case of a 52-year-old woman with worsening IBM who pursued a modified ketogenic diet for 1 year. Adverse effects were mild and resolved 3 weeks into the diet. Prior to starting her ketogenic diet, despite the use of a walking stick at all times, she was experiencing one to two falls per week as well as swallowing difficulties, musculoskeletal pain, and depression. Moreover, magnetic resonance imaging (MRI) of the bilateral thighs during the year prior to the diet indicated worsening muscle inflammation and a 14% decrease in thigh muscle volume, which corresponded to a 4% decrease in the ratio of thigh muscle to thigh total volume. After 1 year on her ketogenic diet, our patient regained independent walking, and her swallowing difficulties, pain, and depression resolved. She maintained her strength, improved in every test of function, enhanced her quality of life, and lowered her blood Creatine kinase. MRI of the bilateral thighs during the year of the diet indicated stabilized muscle inflammation and a 2.9% decrease in thigh muscle volume, which in the context of diet-induced fat loss corresponded to a sustained 1% increase in the ratio of thigh muscle to thigh total volume. This case is unique in that a ketogenic diet was utilized as the primary treatment strategy for a patient with confirmed IBM, culminating in substantial clinical improvement, stabilized muscle inflammation, and a slowed rate of muscle atrophy. Our patient has remained on her ketogenic diet for over 2 years now and continues to enjoy a full and independent life. https://www.ncbi.nlm.nih.gov/pmc/articles/ PMC7674586/

Dr. Expert responds within minutes.

Thanks for sharing. I had seen the study -- hard to draw much conclusions from a single case study but it is interesting. I think a modified ketogenic diet (like Atkins diet) would be a reasonable approach to try, but I would like to see more evidence before recommending this to patients.

Dr. Daughter agrees to try a modified Atkins. I ignore both and order the ketogenic diet book from Amazon—just to look at. I'll take charge with grace, honesty, and positivity. I make a grocery list and buy from the recommended list.

I plunge into the keto diet on Monday. All diets start on Monday. I'm reading about ingesting lots of meat and fat. Exactly the opposite of my usual diet. I was firmly in the "Eat meat as a treat" camp, and fat was never my friend. Keto encourages putting one tablespoon of MCT (medium-chain triglyceride) oil in my morning coffee. I gag!

Scanning the recipe list, I'm trying to find a dinner—something that beloved husband will not notice as "different." Roasted pork stuffed with ham and cheese. Pigs in Blankets, Bacon & Cheese Fat Bombs, homemade guacamole. Despite the fact that there is an avocado tree on my patio, neither of us eats guacamole.

After three days, I'm not exactly rocking the keto way of life. Besides the bad breath, which made me aware I *was* in "ketosis," as well as being in a bad mood, I felt hungry and unsatisfied. I wasn't into making my own guacamole, and although I like bacon with Sunday breakfast, most nutritionists say processed meat is unhealthy. The recipes, "What you can do with hot dogs"—seriously? This cannot be healthy. Bill thinks I'm losing my mind.

Thus ends my short-lived Keto diet.

Mon, June 14, 2021   At the Airport

Sometimes I wonder if Bill is dealing with the reality of my/our current situation. He insisted on another week in Boston when I was eager to get home to my medical team and my own bed. He has ordered a wheelchair to meet us at Logan Airport. We tear through the airport at record speed—plastic bag with items removed from overweight suitcase (mine) on my lap. Suddenly overcome with horror: what if—say—an old boyfriend, pre-Bill, spots me in a wheelchair? Reality check: Never mind, thirty-plus years later, I probably wouldn't be recognizable even with my new Sassoon haircut and highlights.

I look around, noticing all the other old people in wheelchairs, and reflect on how we used to make jokes about knowing we were on our way back to Florida by the number of wheelchairs meeting the plane. I am now number four in line for boarding. Early on is the only benefit of my newly joined group. Who am I, and how did I get here? And what comes next?

When I was twenty years old, I dropped out of Hunter College in New York to accept what was then the glamorous and sought-after position of airline stewardess (now flight attendant). It was a dream job; I got to travel the world first class and stay in five star hotels for practically nothing. No backpacking was involved. The safety announcement on the airplanes has not changed in the over fifty years since I left the job, but today I find the announcement particularly poignant as they review the emergency procedures. *"Should the cabin experience sudden pressure loss, stay calm and listen for instructions from the cabin crew. Oxygen masks will drop down from above your seat. Place the mask over your mouth and nose. Pull the strap to tighten it. If you are traveling with children, make sure that your own mask is on first before helping your children or anyone nearby."*

With crystal clarity, a gong goes off and it's suddenly clear to me how this relates to my new everyday life. It's time to take care of me first. Learn to say no to things I don't want to do. Is it possible to de-program myself, to break old habits and develop new ones at this age? Just wondering.

And I'm newly grateful they have a handicapped bar in the bathroom of the Jet Blue A320—a thought my former self never experienced.

Dr. Expert at Hopkins had handed me 18 pages of IBM facts as a departing gift. A harbinger of things to look forward to. Nowhere is it indicated that this disease can be conquered. Instead it is information to "help you with your new reality." What can I tell others sharing my journey about this disease and diagnosis, except "Do yourself a favor and stop googling"? I can't go backward in time. And I'm not going *through* something; it's more like I'm *in some new thing,* trying to figure a way out. I can also tell anyone who cares to listen: "Don't patronize me." I don't want your pity, which usually comes with unsolicited advice. I tell my close friends and family what I am experiencing, but am private enough to not want busy bodies poking in my business and spreading false information over martinis. Yentas need not apply! I will not get caught in the web of what Rona refers to as "Yentaism."

I want my husband and my daughter to be proud of me—so here's to a future of working hard to stay strong, upright, and positive. My biggest fear is losing my independence. I have just spent three weeks maneuvering uneven streets in Boston with the aid of my trekking pole in one hand and my other arm looped through Bill's. Blurry vision not helping. I think back to taking my mother to the airport, traveling alone at the age of 94 to visit my brother in the state of Washington. I tried to convince her that a wheelchair would be beneficial when changing planes might necessitate long distances. She scoffed at the idea at first and finally acquiesced. I'm liking the wheelchair ride to the terminal, by train in Tampa and then to baggage. We made it in record-breaking time, and even Bill had a hard time keeping up with the friendly young attendant.

Wed, June 16, 2021

And so we are home, albeit exhausted from almost four weeks on the road. I am happy to be sleeping in my own bed. With the hope of an imminent drug trial on hold, we are back to our new reality, which includes an uninvited dependence on my part. I can't climb a ladder to change a lightbulb; I'm unable to reach the shelf with the olive oil bottle. These are tasks I always performed without thinking and now I must ask Bill to help with them, and even worse, I have to wait for him to do it! My husband is a confirmed subscriber to the Italian philosophy of "Domani!" Translation: Never change a lightbulb today, if you can put it off till tomorrow, or the next day, or more likely next week. He learned that from spending much of the past twenty years living and working in Florence. Clearly we came away from that experience having adopted entirely different mottos.

Next!

I am a strong kick-ass woman who is the author of six books and numerous newspaper and magazine articles. I've won awards. Most recently I was the only female among five PhDs and MDs to win an outstanding achievement award and be inducted into my high school hall of fame. Seriously, there's now a photo of me hanging on the wall for all of eternity. I've got this!

The motto **"God helps those who help themselves"** emphasizes the importance of self-initiative and agency. The expression is known around the world and is used to inspire people for self-help. The phrase originated in ancient Greece as "the Gods help those who help themselves" and may originally have been proverbial. It is illustrated by two of Aesop's fables, and a similar sentiment is found in ancient Greek drama. Although it has been commonly attributed to Benjamin Franklin, the modern English wording appears earlier in Algernon Sidney's work.

*I don't have to attend every argument
I'm invited to.*

—W. C. Fields

Chapter 20
LESSONS AND RESOLUTIONS

Tues, June 22, 2021 Self-Healing is a Journey

I am feeling empowered; the ball is in my court, so to speak. So here goes. I am not a victim. I can get better or at least maintain. I will work to get over my fear and anxiety.

And I get that I have to figure it out for myself now. As an empowered woman I am able to embrace fear and command control over my anxiety.

The Covid pandemic is on the wane, and people are getting back to travel and socializing—business as usual. For the past year and a half, no one was doing much of anything but hunkering down at home, dressed in comfy sweats, wearing surgical masks in public, and trying to stay safe. The doors are wide open now, which is a problem for me—for us.

Taking it one day at a time and not projecting to future events is not what I usually do. I accept my current limitations, but that doesn't stop me from hoping for a clinical trial in the fall. That said, Bill is now wanting to return to Boston in September to attend his high school reunion and then go on to New York. There's a Cezanne show at MOMA till the end of September.

Health is a state of BEING and I am committed to achieving optimal health, no matter what. It is with this in mind that I tell Bill it is not good for me to go to Boston and/or New York at this time. I tell him he has to make his own decision about how important the trip is to him. He asks if I'll be okay at home alone. Would his response be considered egocentric or androcentric? Next!

We are Not Alone in our New Reality

There are many people, like me, some younger and some older, who are recipients of an unpleasant and often fatal diagnosis. As rocker Peter Frampton said, "IBM is life altering, not life ending." I can survive this. I'll hang in and all will be okay. After Bill's accident, as he lay in a drug-induced haze, wrapped in gauze like a mummy, his arms and legs in splints so as not to move the skin grafts, he stayed positive. He is the most courageous person I've ever known.

Mon, June 28, 2021   Amazon Fashionista

During Covid isolation, when we were unable to venture very far from home, I ordered anything I needed along with what I clearly did not need online. If only we had bought Amazon stock before Covid! For my newly slender body,

I ordered swim shorts from Amazon with the thought of partially covering the now loose skin on my thighs, along with a bikini top in day-glo yellow. It arrived with enhancing foam push-ups giving the illusion of the body I always wanted. At least the one Bill wanted. Victoria's Secret has nothing on me.

Today, we walk on beautiful Lido beach and we go in the gulf (water temperature 85 degrees). Amazing how buoyant the water is, so we stay in and jump around and swim for half an hour. I am fine; even if I fall I can't hurt myself. Bill can't take his eyes off the swim top, which acts as a floatation device for me. Feeling blissful.

Wed, June 30   Summer Setback

Intense pain at biopsy site on left bicep awakens me in early dawn. It is red, swollen, and throbbing. Take photo and send to surgeon. He says it looks like bacterial infection and to wash with antibacterial soap, but if does not improve go to a local doctor. I am surprised because the incision seemed to be healed after five weeks. But on further investigation I see a couple of dissolvable stitches poking through. Next day is worse so on to urgent care facility, where it is diagnosed as cellulitis infection. I am put on a ten-day heavy-duty protocol of antibiotics. I learn from the doctor that many of the Gulf of Mexico beaches are full of harmful bacteria, sewage spills and such. I google and find the NO-SWIM advisory ban has been posted on local area beaches. Who knew? I grew up thinking saltwater heals everything.

The Statute of Repose vs the Random Exit

When Bill was riding as a passenger in the Lincoln Town Car on that fateful trip from Tampa airport to our home in Sarasota, the car lost its brakes and caught on fire. Bill dove out the window of the speeding car onto Interstate 75 and miraculously survived.

I was told by the State Trooper that the vehicle he was riding in was thirteen years old, which meant that there was no liability by the manufacturer because of the "Statute of Repose." It turns out that twenty states have enacted Statutes of Repose, laws that completely cut off manufacturers' liability for defects once the product reaches an arbitrary chronologic age assigned by the state legislature. In Florida it is twelve years. Who knew that the shiny black Lincoln with the big trunk was thirteen years old? These sedans all looked the same to us.

I'm beginning to think the statute works the same way with health. At a certain age we all have something wrong with us, and the manufacturer, our creator, is no longer responsible. At age 77, my next BIG birthday will be eighty (if I'm lucky), and eighty is not the new sixty. I can attest to that. It seems only a short time has passed since I gathered all of my five brothers and their wives and children to celebrate my father's eightieth when I was newly married and living on the beach in Sarasota, Florida.

One month ago a dear cousin was diagnosed with stage 4 pancreatic cancer and was gone in a month at age 66. Today, we learn that our beloved brother-in-law has been diagnosed with Alzheimer's at age 72. Whoever said that life is fair or that everything happens for a reason? Neither of these is true.

Bill looked at me as I awoke this morning and said in his usual cheerful manner, "You can't die. Can you imagine the line of women at the front door every day—fighting over me? You used to call them the casserole brigade."

I do not like the term caretaker. I prefer to think of my husband as my lover and friend and helper when I need him. Spousal re-education when needed. Every day is a reminder to enjoy every moment. Never forget that!

A Few Words about Conflict and Confrontation

I hate conflict and make every effort to avoid it at all costs. My idea of conflict resolution is to shut my mouth, close my eyes, and hope it goes away. I'm afraid of conflict. But by not arguing a point calmly and intelligently, I give in and end up hating myself for being such a wimp—practicing self-loathing of the highest order.

So here's what I am learning: When you kick the victim mindset to the curb and start thinking like an empowered self-healing dissident, you'll get totally clear on what you need to do to shift your body from sickness to health.

You'll be able to focus on your goals and get busy creating the health and life of your dreams. You refuse to let others dictate what you do but begin to live life on your terms.

You begin to change impossible into "I'm possible" and recognize that whatever you can fathom in your mind, you can create in your life. You begin to love yourself wholeheartedly and are committed to being your true self un-apologetically.

Once you start thinking like an Empowered Self-Healing Fighter you'll start acting like one too.

I have IBM But it doesn't have me, as my nurse friend from Hopkins told me. No one has power over you unless you give it to them—or, as in my case, to it. Whatever control you feel someone or something has over you is because you granted it to them at one point or another.

Resetting Your Buttons

As you reprogram your negative thoughts and learn some positive strategies, you will shift your life. Let go of the past, and constantly purge any leftover self-pity. That stuff just drains your energy. I have to remind myself daily—and sometimes more than once—to *Put yourself first*. You're the number one priority now, and you have to take care of yourself. But there is no room for "Poor Me." Maybe I should make a tee shirt that just says: *"ME* ME."

Resolutions:

I will try hard to reprogram my subconscious mind.

Learn to forgive. Oops! Here comes my mother again. Okay, I forgive. My own decline in health and physical capabilities and writing about it has given me a fresh perspective. I have a deeper understanding and appreciation of my mother. It has made ageism and loss of independence much clearer to me. I have more compassion for what she was going through and the fact that she was without my father for comfort.

Learn to say "No." I do, but then Bill tries to convince me otherwise. Say it again!

In sickness and in health, we should all focus on the love, joy, and gratitude in our life.

Important Lessons

- I have great power within me.
- Understanding my body—how it moves and operates, and how to respect its needs—has helped me to center myself, increase strength and confidence.
- Energy Conservation: Listen to your body and rest when needed.
- Set and maintain your boundaries. I have learned to say **"no"** when I do not want or feel up to doing something. And all was okay when I did!
- Set and maintain your attitude: Go with the flow and hope for the best.
- Make the necessary adjustments to your environment. I have needed to adapt to physical and mental needs that arise as a result of my disease; to prepare our home for safety, e.g., removing throw rugs to prevent slips and falls.
- Use a cane or trekking stick outside for fall prevention.
- Exercise to prevent further deterioration of affected muscles.
- Eat a healthy diet.

- Make social adjustments as needed. For example, we no longer go out to dinner our usual five nights a week. Two evenings works best and in small groups—one or two couples.
- Every morning give thanks for the good things in your life—like waking up.
- Take nothing for granted.
- Understand and be compassionate to your partner, who may not want to face your reality.

What We Can Do Going Forward:

DO

- **Live your life; don't analyze it**. This according to our 93-year-old friend Joseph.
- Stick with the lifestyle changes that work for you in your current situation. They are all interconnected. Don't jump from yoga one week to green drinks and tai chi the next. Find a plan and stick with it. Get your team in place.
- Be a survivor and a fighter. Remember that everybody is different, and each disease works differently depending on the person and their individual lifestyle.
- Be the healthiest, mentally and physically, that you can be.
- Definitely let go of any fear and anxiety. Find a way, or it will eat you up.

- Be patient. Be grateful: make a list of what you are grateful for. Do it again.
- Continually adapt to the physical and mental needs that arise as a result of your diagnosis. Make sure you get accurate information from the best sources. (No random Googling.)
- Let go of things that don't matter.
- Deal with events on a day-to-day basis.
- Detach from people who are no longer a positive force in your life or who are harmful or toxic. It's not easy, but you will be so much happier.

DON'T

- Don't let a diagnosis define who you are. You are not your diagnosis!
- Don't wallow in self-pity.
- Don't dwell on the past.
- Don't fear the future or you will lose today.
- Don't ever, ever give up!

To live in the past is to die in the present.

—Bill Belichick

Chapter 21
DECISIONS

Sun, August 1, 2021

This morning Bill and I are discussing what could be the impending drug trial. We've been told those recruited for the possibility of being a participant will be notified mid-August, and the trial will begin in September, requiring a return trip to Johns Hopkins in Baltimore.

Unbeknownst to each other we have each been doing research, reading reports regarding the trial drug for Sirolimus. I am thinking that Bill is going to be disappointed if I do not want to participate. Serious discussion ensues. We compare notes on success rates of the drug and side effects. It turns out that we are both on the same page.

We go to the exercise equipment store and order a recumbent bike. Then we go to Libby's Brasserie for a late lunch and a glass of wine. I am happy for this day.

Tues, August 3, 2021

I ask Dr. Z, my acupuncturist, his opinion about the possible Sirolimus drug clinical trial. He vehemently opposes me taking it. He is very familiar with the drug, which has been around since the 1990s as a means of staving off rejection for patients with kidney transplants. His daughter took it at age seventeen. "It's a very strong drug and not for you."

So that is final and agreed upon. No participation in the trial should I be called. And there is no guarantee of that, even though I donated three biopsies at the time of surgery. There are three Susan Mice running around now with my muscle.

Thurs, August 5, 2021

It's my birthday. I start the day with a walk around the bay with the good husband. At 11 I go to Pilates, where Marcie presents me with a chocolate, chocolate chip bundt cake, wrapped beautifully with card and balloon. Marcie is fifty, gorgeous, and does not have one lump or bump on her perfect toned body. Off to a great start.

Next stop is Rona, who I have not seen for three weeks. Our topic today covers it being my choice as to what I will focus on. Mainly don't stay focused on pain, neuropathy, and trauma. Live with it; it doesn't define you. This suddenly seems to sink in and make sense. Back to living.

What can I realistically expect? Happiness and gratitude for today and for what really matters. "No one is promised tomorrow."

Mon, August 16, 2021

We have decided to list our home that we never intended to be our "terminal housing." What started as a two-year rental to see if we liked living downtown in a condo turned into a purchase and twenty-two years in our beautiful condo and loving downtown Sarasota on the water. I just hope I have the energy for a move.

I think that if I throw out stuff little by little, the job will not overwhelm me. Yesterday, I started on one part of our combined closet and already have three bags for Goodwill. Today I go into the office closet, where I have shoved just about everything from an overload of framed photos, tapes, and videos of grandchildren to extra pillows and linens. Where to start?

I reach up to a shelf where I have stored folders holding my mother's documents, which include: social security papers, hospital notes, move to assisted living, numerous articles I have cut from newspapers and magazines about senior drivers and how to get them to surrender their license, and on and on. There is the death certificate. There are notes and prayer cards from relatives and friends dating from when she died, poems written by my father, an inventory of what she had brought to Assisted Living.

My mother had recorded her dating events with my father from the day they met at a Halloween dance in 1937, when she was eighteen years old and he was twenty-one. I unfold the well-worn piece of lined paper. Something about reading this dislodges an internal button I didn't know existed.

A guttural howl erupts from the very depth of me like I have never heard before—air pushing out from my lungs, my vocal cords vibrating. A pain so deep and complicated. I drop to a chair and sob uncontrollably. I was so caught up in being pissed off at this woman, then taking care of her, all the while her resisting; moving her, doing for her, helping her, that when she finally died, I swung right into the next phase of informing the relatives, writing the obituary, planning the cremation, the funeral mass, and reception; I never even cried. It's not so much a missing feeling as a longing. I had never grieved the loss of a mother. Until now, three years and four months later. How strange. How sad.

I take this lump of raw emotion to Rona. She is not shocked. I tell her of the cards and notes of sympathy exonerating my "sweet mother" who was so loved by so many.

"The notes invalidated your reality. Did anyone say, 'I'm so sorry for the loss of your mother—she was such a bitch?'" Not a one! Rona says this was pent-up grief on "time release." Now it's over. Some people take thirty years to grieve, she says. I still feel bad that I was not there holding her hand when she passed to another place. I was on the way when Hospice called and told me. Bill and I continued the drive, and I asked them not to touch her before we arrived.

When we got there, I thought we were in the wrong room. I stood in wonder as to why I was so terrified of this little old lady. She was collected and private and never affectionate. I kissed her already cool face and touched her hands—folded over each other, rosary beads interwoven around her fingers. She did not look like my mother.

This was the ultimate transition, but it would be my challenge to let go of the anger and resentment I'd been holding on to. The negative emotions had to go; that whole mind-body connection had activated my current situation to begin with. I was now free but confused. Would I be able to heal on my new journey?

Thurs, August 26, 2021

I can continue the use of creatine powder prior to my exercise routine in hopes of building muscle. I am thinking if I can only get my ankle more stable and focus on the neuropathy, I will be in a good place.

Today I meet with a new ankle and foot Doc, and he x-rays my left ankle. He asks why I never had an MRI. I wondered the same thing, but the original podiatrist who treated the issue almost two years ago said it was unnecessary; that soft tissue damage "will heal itself." So now I am scheduled for an MRI of my left ankle, hoping I can get better mobility, and will meet on Tuesday with a referral for the neuropathy. No one knows the cause of the neuropathy. Medical doctors universally agree there is no effective treatment or cure.

Fri, September 3, 2021

I am starting to bore myself. Here's the deal. MRI shows damaged and stretched out ligaments, along with scar tissue from old injury which was never treated. Dr. suggests surgery; recovery includes wearing a boot up to my knee for six weeks and using crutches. Me: "I'm a slow healer and too old to go through surgery." Cute Doctor, who glances at the computer to see my age. "Well, it says you're 78 but you're not 78. I see people in their fifties who aren't in the shape you're in." Me: "I have Inclusion Body Myositis and I need to exercise and not have a boot on. I'd probably kill myself with the crutches. I have muscle degeneration in my legs."

This is followed by the suggestion of an alternative, less invasive regenerative treatment—an injection of some form of embryonic stem cells from Poland. (I'm not kidding.) This would be in addition to physical therapy and wearing a sports brace.

Could this be the miracle weak ankle cure? It may not be covered by insurance, he tells me, but they will submit it to see if Medicare and Blue Cross are willing to pay the hefty fee of around $5,000 for the injection.

I come home and Google the suggested injection treatment—Wharton's Jelly—to see if it is FDA approved. Sure enough, it comes right up in the browser. Nope, it's not approved. So there's little chance of it being covered by insurance. I read:

> One of the crazier trends in the already completely out of control birth tissue/fake stem cell sales industry is the idea that Medicare now magically covers these products. Of course, none of this is remotely true and all of it comes with federal prison time, but that hasn't stopped many companies from making this claim. Hence, today we'll review the claims of a company called Regenative Labs who has jumped

into that fray. Let's dig in.

Well, enough said. No miracle is about to happen.

Here's what I have learned—again, over and over:

- I am still Susan. My identity is not my illness.
- Adjust to the new reality and don't be pissed off.
- Accept the observable changes. It's a challenge.
- Navigate the new normal. Adapt to the physical and mental needs that are arising.
- The difference between being assertive vs aggressive (attack). It's a rational act.
- Don't let old garbage interfere. Sweep it away.
- Don't be mad at yourself for feeling the way you feel. It's normal to feel these feelings after trauma, loss.and just plain disappointment."Why did this happen to me?"
- "What did I do to deserve this?"
- "I miss my old life."
- Once you recognize these feelings of loss and sadness, you can move to the next step—which is ACCEPTANCE.
- Accept the beautiful parts of what life was before. How wonderful you got to experience such love!
- Stay in the PRESENT moment.

What goodness do you experience in your current life? What sort of feelings do you feel now? Gratitude, love, proud, empowered—what else? You are a survivor. Be grateful for what you do have. On a bad day, it is not uncommon for me to yell out loud. "Okay, I'm fucking grateful that I am still standing!"

I Know What The Answer Is.

I have traced the origin of my stress and anxiety to the painful experiences and traumas in my life. It tells me that our personal reaction to a situation determines the effect that particular situation has upon each person. You can probably say that emotions influence or cause every human ailment. Studies have shown consistently that mind and body are inseparable.

We have the power within us to decide our reaction to life's events, as Viktor Frankl explains in his bestselling book, *Man's Search for Meaning,* with its descriptions of life in Nazi death camps and its lessons for spiritual survival.

I likely could have avoided my chronic illness diagnosis just by having a better and more forgiving attitude towards my mother or perhaps just a better sense of humor.

Panic Disorder

I have experienced anxiety disorder in the form of panic attacks in the past that trigger a "fight-or-flight" response. This did not occur often, but it happened on occasion. Once, when I was sitting in the chair of a new hair colorist, she removed the tinfoil from what were supposed to be fine highlights: orange tiger stripes appeared. My heart pounded seemingly out of my chest, and I started to sweat intensely. Another trigger for me was appearing on TV as an "expert" for one of the books I authored. I had an overwhelming fear that I was going to be asked something I did not know the answer to and make a fool of myself in front of millions of people. On one show, I said to the cameraman "I'm a nervous wreck and my knee is jumping." His response: "Don't worry, only about forty million people are going to be watching you."

Since I have been challenged with IBM, I find when I get into a social situation with more than, say, ten people, I feel dizzy and can't hear. I also think I'm going to just fall over. I can actually picture myself falling to the floor. I experience intense physical and psychological symptoms that can include chest pain and fear of losing control. Basically, my body chemicals become imbalanced. It is a level of discomfort so intense that I feel better staying at home.

But I have learned that stress triggers anxiety, and I realize the only thing I can control is me: My happiness is up to me. I know I need to find inner peace and work on healing everything I can that affects my attitude. I can control stress and listen to my body when it screams for rest. I have stopped focusing outwardly on the possibility of drug trials and miracles. I need more positivity in what is happening now. Our lives are not just about the journey, but who you meet along the way, and I am so fortunate to have Bill in my life.

I cannot say whether things will get better if we change; what I can say is they must change if they are to get better.

—Georg C. Lichtenberg

Chapter 22
FOREVER FLORENCE!

Wed, September 29, 2021 Go Forth and Conquer

We are waiting to hear from the doctors at Johns Hopkins regarding any forthcoming new clinical drug trials for IBM, since Bill, Dr. Z and I have all vetoed Sirolimus. Covid has stalled much research and at the moment there is nothing in the works. Today Bill and I looked at each other in frustration: "Fuck it! Let's just go to Florence!" he says. We also make the significant decision to not sell our condo. We love where we live.

I am now walking with an ankle brace on my left foot—which "fits nicely into a sneaker" according to the foot doc—as well as using a cane. Where am I mentally in all of this? It takes a day for Bill to convince me that we will walk together arm-in-arm over the cobblestone streets and I will be okay. Might as well live our life…carefully!

I spend the next few days on the phone with international airlines—on hold mostly—and then with American Express and online, gathering itineraries and fares. This process takes a full week, but finally success comes with AMEX and a two-for-one fare, and I can use our accumulated miles to end up with a great deal in business class.

Next challenge is finding a place to stay in the ancient city: one that has an elevator and no stairs. It's all in the interpretation. I ask, "Is there a lift?" and when the proprietor says yes, I book a small apartment for three weeks on the sixth floor. Reality hits when I view the online photos and see the low toilet that I cannot possibly get up from. I email the hotel and ask if they can get me a raised toilet seat or tell me where I can buy one, as I have a muscle issue and have difficulty climbing stairs and getting up from a chair.

Communicating with my limited Italian and her better English, we find out that there is indeed a lift to the fifth floor (this is a 700-year-old renaissance palazzo—elevators came much later) but then there are nineteen stairs to "our apartment" on floor six. "Can you manage that?" Ahhhh, no!

Back to square one with accommodations. Bill tells me not to stress, that all will work out okay. Two days later the manager emails that a lovely apartment has opened up on the fifth floor. Slightly more expensive, but newly renovated. She will get a raised toilet seat. No worries! Life is good!!!!!

Where There's a Way—the Special People

It is not a problem getting a wheelchair at Tampa International Airport. In fact, Bill loves the benefit that we are first to board through the jetway. The 8 ½-hour flight on

Delta is from Atlanta to Amsterdam Schiphol Airport—a very large and busy airport. All works well, and I am met with a wheelchair. But a smaller aircraft will be taking us to Florence, and herein lies the problem. There are numerous winding stairs to a bus that arrives in the middle of the tarmac and too many stairs to climb in order to board. The agent tells us that help is on the way.

Minutes pass, and sure enough, two husky guys looking like "incredible hulks" arrive wearing day-glo orange vests, and they make an announcement: "Where are the special people? Please identify yourselves." Bill and I stand around, oblivious until we realize that everyone is looking at us, and that WE must be the referenced "Special People," so we raise our hands frantically like schoolchildren who want to be chosen. The big men take me in a wheelchair, dashing through the terminal and up and down elevators, Bill doing his best to keep up. We are wheeled into the back of a truck, and once inside they clamp the wheelchair safely to the floor, drive to the airplane, and a hydraulic lift transports me up to the catering door. They bang on the door, which a flight attendant opens, and he announces he is delivering the "special people." This worked perfectly, and when we arrived in Florence, the exact method was used in our deplaning. So, yes, I am extremely grateful. A former flight attendant at age twenty who loved her then-glamorous job is now boarding planes a different way. But whatever it took, we made it back to our beloved Florence. I want to kiss the ground.

Florence is the same; I am not. But I am thankful for

the opportunity to be here, back in our second home for over twenty years. "What's the company line?" Bill asks as we slowly navigate, me with the cane and the obvious inability to climb the smallest stairs. We decide on "A little muscle issue and twisted ankle." It all sounds cheery and recoverable. Who knows! Maybe it will be. *Never give up on science. Stay positive!*

Don't be afraid, be mindful and careful!

The second week of our newly adaptable vacation, we are getting a bit relaxed as we cross the rocky Santa Trinita, one of the many bridges over the Arno. It's a challenge, as it is a bit of a hike up and over, but the ultimate situation occurs when we reach the other side and attempt to get past a congested group so we can access the lower step down to the street. I have my cane in my right hand and Bill hanging on to my left. A group of six or so adults with a baby carriage are clustered by the only part of the sidewalk I am able to descend. Bill is saying excuse us, "Scusi" in Italian, and trying to navigate past them, but is largely ignored as we continue to try.

Before I know it, I'm down—not a crash because he is holding me, but definitely down, and it is the first official fall in two years. Absolutely devastating! I am so pissed off. The man comes over and asks me if I am okay (in Italian). I wanted to scream at him, but I do not. The women continue their nonsensical chatter and never look in my direction. It takes a while to see how bad it is and what hurts. I had braced myself with my right forearm, which hurts, and upon inspection is already showing a bruise. But my left ankle, encased in the new brace, is uninjured.

I recover the next day. I want to meet my girlfriends for an aperitivo prior to dinner, as we always did, but I am afraid to go alone walking. Bill escorts me to the Hotel Helvetia & Bristol outside bar and leaves me with my two pals. Brenda has had cancer and was given two months to live by a Florence doctor, who told her to get her papers in order. This was three years ago. She had been diagnosed with metastasized colon cancer that had spread to her liver. Yet here she was, smiling and looking healthy and beautiful. We order drinks, which arrive along with an array of gorgeous appetizers.

Following the diagnosis, Brenda had returned to her native Los Angeles for a second opinion. After days of tests and MRIs, the doctors told her, "Brenda, you have a problem." Her response: "No, doc, I have a condition. You have a problem because you have to fix it!" She befriended her team and told them if they saved her, she would take them all to Florence. And they did, and she had taken the medical team to Florence as promised. Sitting here in the moment with the three of us, like the old days, felt so normal and happy and hopeful. What a joy.

Life is a great and wondrous mystery, and the only thing we know that we have for sure is what is right here right now. Don't miss it.

—Leo Buscaglia

Fri, November 5, 2021

Home again, I continue my *Diagnosis Diaries* and send a draft of the manuscript to my former agent to test the waters. Her response:

Dear Susan,

I just did some research on IBM, and soldiering on with your husband's encouragement and your own caution and fortitude seem like the best route.

As for whether or not to write about it, of course you will; you are a writer. The marketability is restricted not by your Everywoman status but by how very few women (and men) IBM impacts.

My guess is you will come up with an angle that will appeal to a broad audience, with IBM being the first spark for inspiration. So many beautiful, powerful women in our age group who are (literally) brought to their knees in a life-changing moment.

How do we cope when we realize we don't have the health, beauty, or power anymore as we used to define them? How do we battle against invisibility? Where do we find our power, strength, and relevance?   J

The mysterious process of diagnosis gets me thinking about all the OTHER physical ailments and conditions that have no known cause and/or cure. According to the CDC's National Center for Chronic Disease Prevention, "six in ten adults in the US have a chronic disease, and four in ten have two or more." These include ALS, Alzheimer's, MS, glioblastoma, chronic fatigue syndrome, Parkinson's, chronic lung or kidney disease, numerous cancers, heart disease, and many more. That's three out of five adults!

And Tessa Miller, in her book *What Doesn't Kill You: A Life with Chronic Illness,* writes:

"Yet there remains an air of shame and isolation about the topic of chronic sickness. Millions must endure these disorders not only physically, but also emotionally, balancing the stress of relationships and work among the ever-present threat of health complications."

So how do you cope? You have to take charge and manage the disease instead of letting it rule you.

Googling again, I find an article from Harvard Medical School Publishing that seems so helpful I reproduce it here (https://www.health.harvard.edu/staying-healthy/10-steps-for-coping-with-a-chronic-condition):

10 helpful strategies for coping with a chronic condition

- **Get a prescription for information.** The more you know about your condition, the better equipped you'll be to understand what's happening and why. First direct your questions to your doctor or nurse. If you want to do more in-depth research, ask them about trusted sources of medical information on the Web.

- **Make your doctor a partner in care.** We'd put this one more bluntly: Take responsibility for your care, and don't leave everything to your doctor. One way to do this is to listen to your body and track its changes. If you have hypertension, learn to check your blood pressure. If your heart has rhythm problems, check your pulse. For heart failure, weigh yourself every day and chart your symptoms. This kind of home monitoring lets you spot potentially harmful changes before they bloom into real trouble.

- **Build a team.** Doctors don't have all the answers. Seek out the real experts. A nurse might be a better resource for helping you stop smoking or start exercising. You'll get the best nutrition information from a dietitian.

- **Coordinate your care.** In an ideal world, the specialists you see for your heart, your diabetes, and your arthritis would talk with each other every now and then about your medical care. In the real world, this doesn't usually happen. A primary care physician can put the pieces together to make sure your treatments are good for the whole you.

- **Make a healthy investment in yourself.** Part of the treatment for almost any chronic condition involves lifestyle changes. You know the ones we mean — stopping smoking, losing weight, exercising more, and shifting to healthier eating habits. Although these steps are sometimes relegated to the back burner, they shouldn't be. The people who make such changes are more likely to successfully manage a chronic condition than those who don't. Investing the time and energy to make healthy changes usually pays handsome dividends, ranging from feeling better to living longer.

- **Make it a family affair.** The lifestyle changes you make to ease a chronic condition such as high cholesterol or heart disease are good for almost everyone. Instead of going it alone, invite family members or friends to join in.

- **Manage your medications.** Remembering to take one pill a day is tough; managing 10 or more is daunting. Knowing about the drugs you take — why you take them, how best to take them, and what problems to watch out for — is as important as learning about your condition. Talking with your doctor, nurse, or a pharmacist can put drug information into perspective.

- **Beware of depression.** Dark, dreary moods plague a third or more of people with chronic diseases. Depression can keep you from taking important medications, seeing your doctor when you need to, or pursuing healthy habits. Read up on the signs of depression. Let your doctor know if you think you're depressed or heading in that direction.

- **Reach out.** Doctors, nurses, and other health care professionals aren't always the best reservoir for information about what it's like to recover from open-heart surgery or live with heart failure. To get the real scoop, look for a support group in your area and talk with people who have been through what you are facing.
- **Plan for end-of-life decisions.** If the diagnosis of a chronic condition, or life with one, has you thinking about death, channel those thoughts to the kind of care you want at the end of your life. Spelling out whether you want the most aggressive care until the very end, or whether you'd prefer hospice care and a do-not-resuscitate order, can save you and your loved ones a lot of confusion and anguish later on.

Mon, December 6, 2021   Major Setback

If I had a blog, which I don't—because I'm not technically savvy enough to figure out how to do it—you would notice there's been a long hiatus since you've heard any updates or secrets to surviving my diagnosis.

One week after we returned from Italy, I fell, in my own kitchen, and screwed up my right foot pretty badly and broke my big toe. It's the same toe I broke in Florence two years ago. I have lost any recently gained confidence from our successful yet complicated trip to Italy. I am wearing an orthopedic boot with a red sole, not to be confused with Christian Louboutin's trademark color. I'm unable to drive or exercise. This brings with it a distinct loss of security as well as a newly borrowed accessory: The Walker. It feels like I'm dancing the Cha Cha—one step forward and two steps back.

Disclosure to Loved Ones: Martha No More

I don't really know what any of our immediate relatives know about my illness and our life change. Bill is always very positive and tends to downplay the situation, but living it, I can feel my lowered capabilities. We get a call that one of our daughters and family of six are coming for Christmas, and I am happy, but I feel an urgency to let them know that my entertaining skills are on the wane. I decide to put it in writing once and for all and send them an email explaining my diagnosis and current limitations.

Sun, December 19, 2021

Covid seems under control locally and we are all vaccinated and boosted, so we decide to attend one Christmas party of dear friends. We switch the walker for a cane, put the sneakers on, and we're off. We walk in, and I immediately scan for a place for me to sit and not move for the duration. Dutiful, non-complaining husband gets me a glass of sparkling water and some hors d'oeuvres. It's okay once I get there, but the prep work leaves me exhausted: shower, hair, makeup, festive ensemble. At least I'm skinny at 117 pounds—marriage weight. This is something I was not able to achieve in the past ten years—not for lack of trying—but I was great at camouflage.

We declare it was a successful evening, which means we caught up with friends, enjoyed ourselves, and the evening felt "almost normal." After we get home and have the *post mortem*, I head for the closet to hang up my pants and somehow when reaching for the hangar, both knees give out and I am DOWN! On the floor, on my knees, scared, and truly discouraged. "I give up," I say to Bill as he lifts me under my arms and pulls me to a standing position.

My head on the now damp pillow, he whispers in my ear, "We never give up. You're with Superman, remember?" *What would I do without him?*

Wed, December 22, 2021

I want to go out for Christmas dinner. Bill insists on entertaining at home. I am on a walker with a broken foot. We compromise. I hire someone to come in and cater the dinner with family. It's not Martha, but it works.

Well, sort of. Pat, a referral from a close friend, was the only available "service person" in Sarasota on Christmas Day. Turns out she was planning on divorcing her husband and wanted to get out of her house soon after opening presents with her children on Christmas morning. I was the lucky recipient and she would come at noon. Did I need her to bring anything? I said, "No, thank,you, unless you'll be anywhere near Morton's Gourmet Market and can pick up some paper-thin, freshly sliced prosciutto for my charcuterie board."

This seemed to really excite Pat. "C h a r c u t e r i e, nice," she said slowly, and the way she pronounced it sounded sinister. I had pre-ordered a tenderloin roast and side dishes, along with tons of food for the appetizers. Pat arrived carrying a supermarket bag with an array of pre-sliced and pre-packaged salami and thick-sliced prosciutto. She was seriously excited about adding this stuff to my otherwise perfect food board, and she kept touching and moving all the food.

"Don't touch the food," I said, a little too snarky, to which she replied, "I'm only arranging the *charcuterie*" in that creepy low tone. No one noticed but me, of course.

Fri, December 31, 2021

In the two to three years since the onset of this mysterious disease called IBM that has left me on a walker with a broken foot and unstable with progressively weakening muscles, and exhaustion, the doctors do not have the answers and offer no treatment. I will become my own researcher and scientist and will keep my eyes open for anything that can help. I have to heal myself.

The specialists tell me there is nothing I can do but exercise, but not too much. Life-changing, life-saving treatments do not exist at this time. But a tremendous amount of research continues. There will most likely be additional clinical trials in the future—new uses for existing prescription drugs—but that has not happened. At least I have a diagnosis. I would like to have my former life back, and then I could possibly take what I've learned and be able to help others. I feel the responsibility to get things in order. But I'm not giving up--I was born August 5. Leos are lions. They are determined and fierce. This is my life now and I intend to stay positive and live it to the fullest—joyful and hopeful.

I give you these words of inspiration from fellow New Jersey native Bruce Springsteen, who spoke of his mother's decade-long struggle with Alzheimer's disease:

"Remember that the future is not yet written, so when things look dark, do as my mighty mom would insist: Lace up your dancing shoes, get out on the floor and get to work."

Today was eight weeks post- toe-break and walker. I drove for the first time—to acupuncture. Getting back on the schedule. Life is good.

Bye Bye Botox

I used to worry about getting old, gaining weight, thinning hair, lines around lips. Now I want to get old. I embrace the wrinkles. Oh, the silly fixations on aging and the accompanying lines and wrinkles! I considered a tiny line around the eyes a flaw. Something to get rid of.

I've been doing Botox injections since my TV book tours started for my second book, *Why Men Commit*. That's years of temporarily paralyzing a few facial muscles between my eyebrows. I never read the side effects, nor did I experience any—or so I thought. But in looking through a magazine recently, I come across an ad for Botox Cosmetic, which points to the fact that indeed there can be side effects and states clearly that we should read the Warnings.

The warnings:

BOTOX® Cosmetic (onabotulinumtoxinA) is a prescription medicine that is injected into muscles and used to temporarily improve the look of moderate to severe forehead lines, crow's feet, and frown lines between the eyebrows in adults.

-

Talk to your doctor about BOTOX® Cosmetic and whether it's right for you. There are risks with this product - the effects of BOTOX® Cosmetic may spread hours to weeks after injection causing serious symptoms. Alert your doctor right away as difficulty swallowing, speaking, breathing, eye problems or muscle weakness can be a sign of a life-threatening condition. Patients with these conditions before injection are at the highest risk. Side effects may include allergic reactions, neck and injection-site pain, fatigue and headache. Allergic reactions can include rash, welts, asthma symptoms, and dizziness. Don't receive BOTOX® Cosmetic if there's a skin infection. Tell your doctor your medical history, muscle or nerve conditions (including ALS/Lou Gehrig's disease, myasthenia gravis, or Lambert-Eaton syndrome), and medications, including botulinum toxins, as these may increase the risk of serious side effects.

Well, I do have a muscle and nerve condition. In further reading I find that the product can travel to damaged muscles and is excreted through the liver and kidneys, and can cause a "life-threatening condition." I am obviously of high risk.

Fuck! I wonder if all the years of doing this have triggered my current condition. Too late now. My only choice is to stop the injections forever. *What if my face collapses?*

I immediately email my specialist at Johns Hopkins with this information, which can be helpful to other women. Are other women with chronic illnesses still vain like me? Regardless, I must bid a sad goodbye to an old friend that always made me look and feel better.

January 2022   Rona

Me: I was looking through a magazine, and there was an ad for Botox Cosmetic. **Warning: Read this.** And there it was in plain sight, after years of Botox injections every six months in a successful attempt to rid myself of frown lines caused by concentrating and writing for hours. For me it was a miracle. Maybe the warnings were there all along, but I don't think so.

Rona: Learn to love your lines and wrinkles. Accept and embrace them. You don't need Botox.

I tell her the story of my dermatologist insisting that I do some fillers a few years ago. As I was sitting in her chair, hoping she would not find yet another basal cell skin cancer, she looked and me and said, "I've been begging you for five years to let me inject something into those lines around your mouth. They are the only aging part of your face." I said, "How much is it?" And she tells me and says it will make a huge difference in my appearance. So I ask if there are any side effects. None! By the time I arrived home I had extreme bruising on either side of my mouth. I looked like Fu Manchu without the mustache. She wanted to inject the upper lip as well, but I wouldn't let her—if I had, I would have had a total Fu Manchu. Frankly, after $600, the only difference I saw was severe bruising that even camouflaged with half an inch of Cover-up, was very obvious.

Rona: Women are doing too much of these fillers. It's dysmorphic disorder—they think they look good with chipmunk cheeks and puffed out lips. You need to *love* who you are!!

Forces beyond your control can take away everything you possess except one thing, your freedom to choose how you will respond to the situation.

—Viktor Frankl, *Man's Search for Meaning*

Chapter 23
A NEW YEAR

Stay the Course

I am focusing on knowing as much as possible about my disease, as well as identifying the leaders in the field. I've already been to three of the leading specialists. I hope that with all the Covid research, someone will find a cure for IBM. I read about a scientist at MIT who is working day and night to find a cure for the muscle disease of his father. I spend a day writing to him and researching, only to find he has moved on to a company in California.

Thurs, January 6, 2022

I did not hear back from the famous scientist. Since there is still no treatment or cure, it's up to me to do the research. I write to another IBM Doctor at UC Irvine.

How did I get here? I credit trauma and stress that my mind could not handle, so it attacked my body, my genes, on a cellular level. Poor sleep, anxiety, toxic diet, toxic environment. My very foundation was compromised.

My first truly traumatic narrative began in 1967 and lasted till 1972, when I was twenty-nine: a youthful five-year marriage to a seemingly charming man who was soon revealed to be a bipolar cocaine addict and domestic abuser and then topped it off by being a deadbeat dad. The economic impact was especially difficult, as I was literally destitute and had to work hard to change that narrative. And for the most part I did change it, by leaving the marriage and focusing on the gift of my two- and three-year-old babies, who were my biggest pride and motivation. I felt empowered! Hatred brings no joy, but living well truly is the best revenge. I was able to forgive myself for marrying Mr. Wrong and move forward. My past made me strong.

Nevertheless, the experience carried with it rumbling aftershocks for me, and even more so for my children. And the responsibility of raising two children on my own was daunting. I found underlying scar tissue decades later, when I was dealing with my mother and not wanting to take on the burden.

There is no longer any question that the effects of stress are cumulative and will catch up to your health eventually. I am in the process of changing my lifestyle and eliminating what broke my immune system in the first place. Am I too old to learn new tactics?

I make a list for myself.

1. Get papers and possessions in order. Whenever I think about my own mortality, I feel a very strong

urge and responsibility to organize and streamline my affairs. I need to feel comfortable knowing my spouse and/or family will be able to deal with things.

2. FIX YOURSELF: Get rid of toxic friends and relatives, toxic diets, and toxic environments.
3. Hang tough. Stay determined and focus on keeping up the fight against your disease.
4. Keep your foundation as healthy as possible.
5. Increase the positivity. Let go of negativity. Shift your mind and shift your life.
6. Stay in the present.
7. Be grateful for what you have.
8. Don't complain No one wants to be around a complainer. Stick to the royal family's unwritten rule of "Never complain, never explain."
9. Believe you can survive this. Have a passion for your future.
10. Take back your power.

And Another List: Some Things I've Learned

1. We're all on the same path, some going faster than others, some richer, some poorer, some healthier than others for longer, but no one escapes the inevitable. It's the final part of life.
2. Inflammation is the cause of most, if not all, diseases. We all know what the culprits are: trauma, stress, poor sleep, toxic diet, toxic environment, and toxic people. Identify whatever

triggers are causing inflammation and eliminate them. You can do it! Lifestyle is about 90% of health; genetics 10%.

3. A serious diagnosis is not necessarily the end. It can actually be a new beginning and your life may change. Go with the flow! Learn to love your changed self.

4. You are responsible for your health. Be your own advocate. It's okay to ask for the accommodations you need in order to do the things you want to do.

5. Do the research, ask the questions. Believe in science and find the experts for your particular disease. Build your best team.

6. Learn to ask for help. It could eliminate a fall or accident. You'll need to learn new tactics for getting what you need, and that may require enlisting the aid and support of others.

7. Program your brain to do an enjoyable activity when you're having a bad day.

8. Practice the art of compassion for the elderly and those struggling with a chronic disease.

9. Rediscover joy and find new purpose.

10. Practice mindfulness. One of the challenges of anxiety is learning how to live in the moment—reprogramming the tendency to constantly be worrying about what happened in the past or what *could* happen in the future.

11. Find new ways to navigate the world.

12. Think of your situation as a challenge rather than a tragedy.

Going Forward: Final Advice

Life is full of surprises sometimes, so hang in there no matter what your circumstances.

You have two ways to go. You can stay home and feel sorry for yourself, or you can live your life and do what brings you joy. Feeling sorry for yourself is not going to fix you.

- Be a person of hope and persevere. Cultivate qualities of optimism, practicality, and independence.
- Become a disability advocate.
- Try to live in a world without boundaries.
- View your condition not as a tragedy, but just the way things turned out.
- Walk through the world joyfully, but carefully.
- Don't let emotional stress convert into physical symptoms.
- You've got to keep going and keep fighting.
- Most importantly, slow down and stay mindful.

I wish you health, happiness, hope, and healing!

The capacity for hope is the most significant fact of life. It provides human beings with a sense of destination and the energy to get started.

—Norman Cousins

AFTERWORD

June 2022   The Emotional Roller Coaster Continues

It's impossible to give up hope and settle for reality. At least for me. It is human nature always to find fresh cause for optimism. People always hope for the best, even in the face of adversity.

Our friend recommends a new "life changing" book by motivational speaker Tony Robbins, written with two Harvard- and MIT-trained MDs and PHD. *Life Force* is an instant bestseller, introducing numerous "miracle cures," some available now, some to be FDA approved in the future—perhaps. After reading the entire book of some 700 pages, I am convinced that I can benefit from stem cell treatment, not yet widely available in the US.

I apply to the Stem Cell Institute in Panama. I have now sold some of my recently inherited stock and would spend the $25,000 (including treatment and hotel), because that is what happens with an illness. One will do anything, and spend any amount, to get their life back. The old slogan "As long as you have your health!" definitely applies, because when you don't have it—that is all that matters!

I fill out a long, tedious online application that includes my age of now 78. After successfully clicking the SUBMIT button, I take a deep breath and sit back. This could be it. With stem cell therapy I can regain my ability to get up from a chair and climb stairs. I would feel stable again, walking with Bill like we always did. Enjoying life, sunshine, and travel!

The site thanks me for the submission and tells me that they will review my application and get back to me in an average time of five days. I'm thinking what my father would say if he knew I'd sold my Exxon Mobil stock to go to Panama: "Are you out of your goddamned mind"?

The next morning, less than 24 hours after hitting submit, my answer arrives:

Dear Susan C Kelley:
Thank you for your interest in the Stem Cell Institute, in Panama City, Panama.

Unfortunately, after reviewing the application you submitted, we regret to inform you that we do not treat your condition. We only treat autism, cerebral palsy, heart failure, MS, osteoarthritis, rheumatoid arthritis, spinal cord injury and some autoimmune diseases (on a case-by-case basis). . . .

If we can be of assistance in the future, please do not hesitate to contact us.

Warm regards,

Medical Staff
Stem Cell Institute
Panama City, Panama

Okay, I am probably saved from making a foolish mistake.

Mon, June 13, 2022   Hope Springs Eternal

We used the opportunity of being in Boston to meet with another IBM expert at Brigham & Women's.

Young, studious, handsome, and serious doc: "What are you looking for?"
Answer, Bill: "Hope."

Doc: "We have developed a new drug specifically for IBM. It is currently being tested for safety in Australia. We could be looking at a clinical trial in three to six months. Hang in there. Progress is being made."
We are happily stunned. The big honcho chief of neurology enters and confirms what the fellow has just told us. There is a fifty/fifty chance of getting the placebo, but I'll take that chance. The doc is optimistic, and I'm hopeful. "Would I be interested in the trial?"

People will keep on hoping, no matter what the odds. As we leave Brigham & Women's, there would be a lilt in my step if my feet would only lift from the ground.

We meet with an ankle surgeon with my MRI in hand, for a second opinion on having the arthroscopic Brostrom surgery for stability on my left ankle. He encourages me to go forward, telling me my ankle is not going to get better, only worse. I will be the Empress of Recovery.

Fri, July 15, 2022   Living In The Now

A year ago, I wasn't sure I would make it to the high school graduations of our two grandsons this June, one in Chapel Hill and the other in Boston—but we did. I missed the family wedding in Maine, as it required a ferry ride and walking on dirt roads. I encouraged Bill to go with his daughters. That's called adapting to the current situation and not taking unnecessary chances.

I'm on the right track.

I have formed healthier relationships and learned to set boundaries.

I have learned to forgive and let go—to focus my energy on forgiving people who have hurt me in some way, from the smallest slight to the most grievous injuries. Forgiveness is letting go of your pain, accepting what happened, and releasing it. Their actions stem from their own damage; but their damage does not have to become mine, or yours. Don't allow the damage done to you by others to shape who you are.

I no longer live in fear and anxiety. I am committed to

achieving optimal health no matter what. I stay aware of what science is offering but understand there is no quick fix.

We are living our best lives and feel empowered. We remain grateful for what we have, for each other, and hope to be walking into our eighties!

I've never had a "Bucket List" because I pretty much did everything I wanted to do. But suddenly I do have a "Bucket Thing." It's kind of weird, but I'd like to learn how to play the ukulele! I can visualize myself playing "I'll See You in My Dreams" and "Somewhere Over the Rainbow." I'm on it. Stay tuned. I think I can do it.

*The secret of change
is to focus all of your energy
not on fighting the old,
but on building the new.*

—Socrates

POSTSCRIPT

August 2022

We have just returned from a wonderful trip to Henley-on-Thames and Ireland. I would say it's most likely my final international trip and one I was determined to make.

I still find it amazing how I have had to adapt from my usual hyper and independent self to a calmer version who takes few chances where safety is involved and has learned to ask for what I need. Everyone has been beyond gracious. Wheelchairs at airports are a must, and it's okay with us.

I am scheduled for left ankle surgery to tighten and reattach the ligaments. Although it will be an unpleasant recovery, wearing an orthopedic knee boot for at least a month it will help with my stability. Then I only need to keep exercising until a drug is available to stop the degeneration. Until then, I am grateful for my amazing team, including Bill; Dr. Z, my acupuncturist; and Marcie, my Pilates instructor. I hope to continue aging-- despite the fact that it will be in sneakers. I might even make eighty!

Oprah on Maya Angelou:
Her greatest lesson—besides her gems of insight and inspiration—is the way she has approached aging, with such acceptance and assurance. Several years ago, when I asked her what it was like to turn eighty, she said, "*Baaaby*, the eighties are hot! You want to try and make it there if you can."

I'm going to end on that note.

Our Epitaph!

***THEY LIVED AND LAUGHED AND
LOVED AND LEFT.***

—James Joyce, *Finnegan's Wake*

And the world will never be the same.

A NOTE ABOUT THE AUTHOR

Susan Kelley is the author of six nonfiction books: *REAL WOMEN SEND FLOWERS, WHY MEN COMMIT, WHY MEN STRAY/WHY MEN STAY, THE SECOND TIME AROUND: Everything you Need to Know to Make Your Remarriage Happy, I OPRAHED, And Other Adventures of a Woman of a Certain Age* and *FOREVER FLORENCE, A Memoir.*

Her best-selling relationship books have been translated into several foreign languages including Japanese, Polish, Dutch and Turkish.

Susan has appeared as guest "relationship expert" on The Oprah Winfrey Show, The Early Show on CBS NEWS, MSNBC, FOX News and numerous other national and local television programs. She is a member of The Author's Guild.

She lives in Florence, Italy and Sarasota, Florida.

www.ingramcontent.com/pod-product-compliance
Lightning Source LLC
Chambersburg PA
CBHW051410250726
48656CB00011B/87